Knots, Knots and More Knots

The Complete Guide Of Knot Making Indoor, Outdoor And Sailing Knots

By: Andrew Williams

Introduction

Chapter 1: Indoor Knots

Chapter 2: Outdoor Knots

Chapter 3: Sailing Knots

Chapter 4: Necktie Knots

Chapter 5: Fisherman's Knots

Chapter 6: Decorative Knots

Chapter 7: Other Knots

Conclusion

Introduction

Knots are an integral part of life for all of us, their use often starts when a young child begins to play basic games with string and then further develops when they learn to tie their shoelaces. We use knots in many areas of everyday life although many people have difficulty constructing even the most basic knots correctly. From the very simple and practical half hitch or square knot to intricate and very fancy decorative knots used in dressmaking, embroidery and leather work. Knots are used in one form or another to join or secure objects in many parts of the home, garden, workshop and office. All types of people at all levels from housewives to surgeons, executives, farmers, shopkeepers, teachers, builders, engineers and sailors all use and make knots. Many children learn how to make basic knots during activities like Boy Scouts and Girl Guides, but for other people this simple skill eludes them.

The earliest evidence found of people using knots dates from about 500,000 years ago, in the form of spherical stones, these, it is thought were most probably used as bola weights when hunting and must have been secured or tied on in some way (i.e. knots). Other evidence of early knots comes from 300,000 years ago with the finding of perforated objects such as beads and pendants dated from about this time. Because of the organic and therefore biodegradable nature of the actual string, rope or cordage used, (hair, wool, sinews, skins and vegetable fibers and the like) no specimens have yet been found.

As wildlife enthusiasts know, wild gorillas that have never been near man are able to make and use complete knots such as "granny" and "reef" knots. This suggests that using and discovering functional knots predated that of using fire and the wheel, basically, knot tying started before the evolution of modern man began.

Well preserved bows and arrows from the Paleolithic area about 24,000 B C have been found that were made using cordage, secured with knots and also from the same era archeologists have found well preserved figurines that show belts made using cords tied with knots that suggests that a variety knots were known during this time period.

Apart from their purely functional uses, knots from early times were used as an important part of the arts of magic, medicine and a large variety of religious activities. There are many cultures who used intricate knot designs to record their history, to tell stories, and for counting or mathematics, as well as for purely decorative purposes.

A good well-made knot can save your life if you're in a survival situation, during a rescue or when performing first aid. A knowledge of knots is essential when securing a load, towing, climbing, lifting weights or working over water, because a poorly made or using the wrong knot can be dangerous as knots can slip or undo causing accidents.

Knots can be made in a multitude of different ways; they are often used to connect 2 or more items together from an endless array of different types of twines, threads, strings, ropes, wires and chains, made from natural items such as cotton, wool, hair, catgut, silk, hemp, flax, animal skins (thongs) as well as many man-made products such as nylon, polyester and metals such copper aluminum, steel, silver gold and other precious metals.

Every culture has its own selection or types of knots that have been used by and passed down from generation to generation. A well-tied knot is often considered to be a true work of art. Some knots have unusual names such as a "hangman's noose" or "wagoneer's hitch" (many people know this as a truckie or truckers knot), these names give you a glimpse into the history of the knot and how they came to be. They can be used with a rope to handcuff a burglar, lasso a steer or make a ladder, mend or fabricate clothing and bedding.

John Smith of Pocahontas and James Town fame published a manual for seamen called "A Sea Grammar" in 1627 which had a section on splicing and knot tying, this manual suggests that a sailor only need to master and rely on 3 knots, The "Sheepshank Knot", the "Wall Knot" and the "Bowline Knot".

This book gives a practical guide to help you to learn how to tie some basic knots safely and securely as well as ideas on how to choose the right rope and knot for the task you have as every experienced outdoors man (and Woman) knows, there are right and wrong knots for certain jobs.

Chapter 1: Indoor Knots

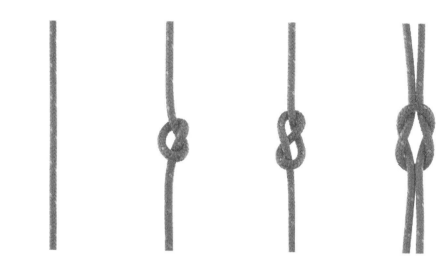

Thumb Knot or Overhand Knot

The thumb knot is one of the simplest types of knot, it can be used to tie off the end of a rope to stop it fraying, to mark off units (place a knot every foot, yard, meter etc) or as a stopper to stop ropes slipping (place the rope through a snug hole and form this knot to prevent the rope slipping back through).

To make the knot;

- Form a loop and pass the end through it and then pull it tight to form the knot.
- If a larger stopper knot is required, the first turn can be followed by a second to create a larger stopper knot, the double stopper knot.

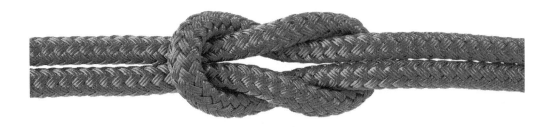

Granny Knot

The Granny knot has many uses around the home, it is the most common knot used. Many people use it to tie their shoe laces, but, as most people will have found, it often comes untied. The solution if you use a granny knot to tie your laces is to make a double knot or 'double your shoelaces". The reason the granny doesn't stay tight and comes undone is because it is not a "balanced" knot. You can tell if a granny knot has been used as the bow will not sit straight, it will sit crookedly instead of across the shoe, it will tend to sit heel to toe.

If you wish to tie your shoelaces or make any sort of bow knot that will not come undone by itself, use the "Reef Knot, Square Knot" (explained next) or "Slipped Reef knot"

To make a Granny Knot

1. Use either 2 cords or 1 long cord
2. Place 1 end of the cord in each hand and lay the right hand cord over the left.
3. And then push it under the left hand cord, forming a half knot
4. Then lay the right hand cord over the left
5. And then push it under the left hand cord, forming the full knot.

6. Pull firmly with equal force on the cords tightening the knot

Right over left and then Right over left again will make this knot.

To make it into a bow

1. After tying the half knot
2. Fold each end to make a loop.
3. Then lay the right hand loop over the left.
4. And then push it under the left hand loop, forming the full knot.
5. Pull firmly with equal force on the loops tightening the knot

The Reef Knot or Square Knot

The Reef knot is often used to tie two cords of equal thickness together where a low strain knot is required. It is easy to tie and undo except when under pressure, but is not suitable for smooth ropesor cords such as nylon. Being an easy knot that is quick to make and convenient, it's popular among sailors, climbers, gift wrappers and homemakers. This knot is usually adequate for most casual applications, but not suitable for heavy loads or in situations where knot integrity is important.

To make the knot

Use either 2 cords or 1 long cord

1. Take the ends of 2 cords and lay the right hand cord over the other (if you wish to lay the left hand cord over the other just reverse all the following instructions)
2. Place the right hand cord under the left hand cord in the same way you would for tying your shoe laces
3. Bring the right hand cord back over the left hand cord (this is called a half knot).
4. Bring the right hand cord over the other rope

5. Push the right hand cord under the other rope
6. Pull firmly with equal force on all four lengths of cord to tighten the knot.

To make a bow (as in tying laces)

1. After tying the half knot
2. Fold each end to make a loop.
3. Then lay the right hand loop over the left
4. And then push it under the left hand loop, forming the full knot.
5. Pull firmly with equal force on the loops tightening the knot

The Larks Head Knot

The lark's head knot is also known as the 'cow hitch', it is very simple and quick to apply. It can be used for attaching just about anything to anything else such as a ring, rod, or even a ribbon. This knot is unique as it can be used with complete loops, like rubber bands or hoops of cordage.

The lark's head knot is often used to start projects such as macramé or plaiting. It can also be used to attach charms to other objects like cell phones, bags etc.

To make the Knot

1. Fold your cord in half, or if using a loop, find the spot on the loop that you'd like to be joined up.
2. Lay the folded cord on the object you're attaching it to.
3. Loop the rest of the line around the object and through the bend and pull tight.

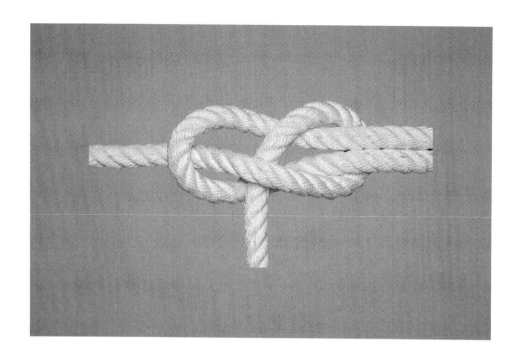

The Weaver's Knot

The Weaver's Knot, Sheet Bend or Becket Knot is a stronger knot than a square knot and often used for joining different size lines. As the name implies, it is used to join broken threads in the textile industry, this knot is also used to make fishing nets and hammocks.

The Boy Scouts rhyme Make a loop in one end. The rabbit goes out of the hole and around the tree, then back under his path.

To make the Knot

1. Create a bight (Any section of line that is bent into a U-shape is a bight) in the end of the cord to be tied.
2. Take the second cord and tug it up through the bight
3. Pass the working end beneath the bight

4. Tuck the working end beneath itself in such a way that both short ends are located on the same side of the completed knot.

The Half Hitch Knot

The half hitch knot is a fairly easy overhand knot. The movable end of the rope is wrapped over and then under fixed part and tightly pulled. Although a complete knot on its own, it is seldom used because it is very insecure, two half hitches together can be used to tie a rope to a tree, boat or any object. In most stances it is used in combination with other knots often for tying any loose end for additional protection and safety.

Because this knot is attractive it is often used decoratively for designs and half hitch whipping.

To tie the Knot

1. Pass the end of a cord around the object you wish to tie, bringing it back to you forming a loop
2. Pass the end of the cord through the loop between the object and yourself forming a knot
3. To make this more secure pass the cord through again in the same direction to make what is called 2 half hitches or a double half hitch.

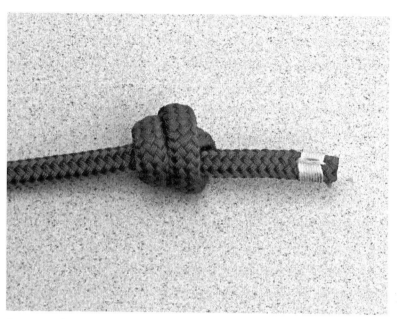

Stopper knots

The stopper knot is mostly used by climbers to prevent the rope from pulling through devices or other knots. It's often used with Bowline and Figure 8 knots and its main advantage is it is easy to tie and very safe. As its name would suggest – the stopper knot stops the rope from slipping through and untying.

To make a Stopper knot:

1. Create a loop
2. Wrap the short end around itself twice
3. Pull it through the loop
4. Tighten the knot equally

5. Secure every additional knot with a stopper knot

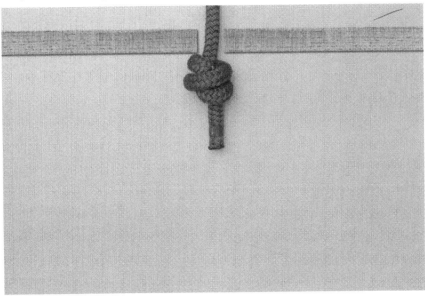

Double Overhand Stopper

The Double Overhand Knot is a stopper derived from the Overhand Knot, simply more reliable and bigger for an additional turn. It's a reasonable extension which makes the knot more challenging to loosen and untie, acting as a simple stopper or even to increase the safety of a second knot.

To make a Double Overhand Stopper:

1. Make sure to take enough rope and make a loop.
2. Pull one end through the loop.
3. Pass it through once more.
4. Tighten it and you have a top stopper knot!

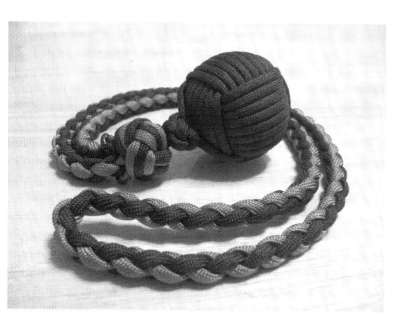

The Monkey's Fist Knot

The Monkey's Fist Knot is mostly used for tying the climbing rope so it could be thrown long distance because it creates a massive end to the rope. The name comes from the shape that you get when you tie the knot. It is the perfect solution for every outdoor sport where the rope is needed to be thrown without coils catching the wind.

To make a Monkey's Fist Knot:

1. Wrap the rope three times around your fist
2. Pull one end through the loops
3. Wrap the rope three times around the set of loops
4. Take the end inside and through the first-made set of loops
5. You should have completed the second set of loops. Wrap them three times inside the first set of loops.
6. Take the end back and make a stopper at the long end.

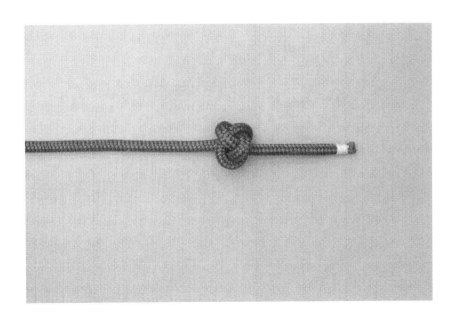

Ashley stopper knot

Ashley stopper knot (also known as Oysterman's stopper) represents probably the best bulky stopper knot. When tightening correctly, at the end of the rope it has the shape of a trefoil. It provides excellent resistance to pulling through the opening than any other knot. It can be multiplied and also it can form a larger knot.

To make Ashley stopper knot:

1. By passing tag end over the standing line you will create a small loop at the bottom of the line.
2. Over that standing line, tie an overhand knot.
3. Make sure that overhand knot is tightened strong enough and then take tag end and pull it through the loop.
4. Tag end needs to go all the way through the loop and knot needs to be slide down tight enough.
5. Make sure both ends are pulled tight.

Chapter 2: Outdoor Knots

Different types of Hitch Knots

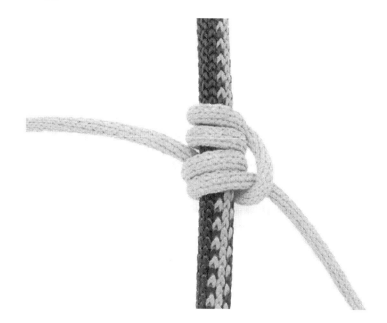

The Blake's Hitch

The Blake's Hitch is a friction type knot popular with arborists for ascending and descending on ropes. This hitch is convenient because it can be tied using the end of a rope or cord.

To tie the Knot

1. Wrap the cord four times around other cord, working it from the bottom to the top.
2. Leave enough room in the 2nd wrap to accommodate the tag end of the rope.
3. Run the tag end down to and over standing line, behind the main static cord and out through the 2nd wrap.
4. Tighten the knot and finish it with a "Figure Eight Knot" for a stopper at the end of the line.

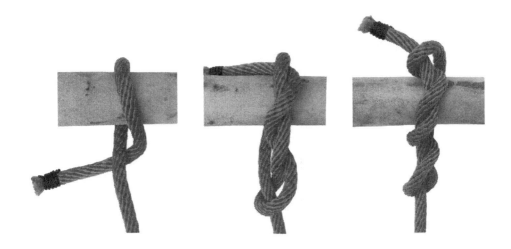

The Timber Hitch

The timber hitch was developed to pull logs and is often used for handling cargo; this hitch performs well under load and almost falls apart when the load slackens. Often when towing a log or pole the hitch is attached in the middle of the log and a half hitch is placed at the end to act as a guide.

This Hitch is the same as the Bowyers knot as it is used by bowmen to attach the end of the bowstring onto a longbow. Guitar and ukuleles also use this hitch for the string attachment.

To make the Knot

1. Pass the working end of your cord around the object you want to haul
2. Turn the cord around itself, the standing part.
3. Tuck the working end back around itself three times inside the loop
4. Make several half hitches near the forward end for use when hoisting and to stop the log from twisting.

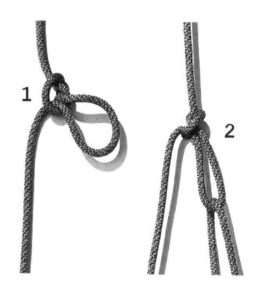

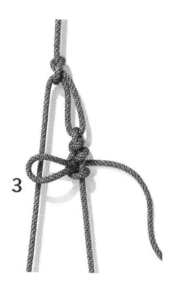

The Trucker's Hitch Knot

The Trucker's Hitch is used to cinch or tie down a load. Using this combination of knots allows a line to be pulled very tight, securing the load. The Trucker's Hitch is probably the most useful hitch there is, it allows loads of many types including heavy loads and loads of uneven shapes to be easily secured in place. Once you have attached the line and used the trucker's hitch to pull the line to the tightness you desire, using a pulley-like effect on the loop in the center of the line, the knot can be secured in place by using a few half hitche knots around both lines or only one end, depending on preference.

To make the Knot

1. First one end of your cord has to be secured to a good tie point
2. About midway on the cord, tie a loose half hitch knot to build a loop in the middle of the rope, ensuring the loop is formed using the loose part of the rope or it may tighten under pressure.
3. Feed the cord around another secure tie point, ensuring it can slip through as it tightens and feed the free end through the loop

4. Using the loop you made in the line as a pulley, pull downward with the free end, making it as tightly knotted as you can and then secure the knot by using two half hitches around both ends of the lines.

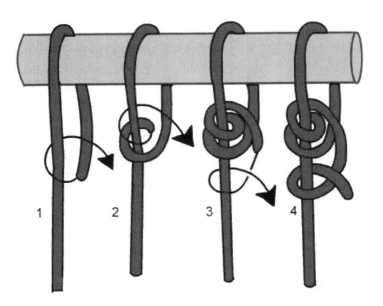

The Taughtline Hitch

The taughline hitch is a rolling hitch tied to a tight line after it has been secured to an object. The knot can be adjusted to loosen or tighten your line, then holds tight under a heavy load. It is very useful for lines that could need to be adjusted making these adjustments easy. It is perfect for tying down a lid or a tent guy line.

To make the Knot

1. First place your cord around a fixed point several feet from the end of your cord
2. Then coil the free end of your cord twice around the standing line working it back toward the fixed point.

3. Wrap the cord around the line just above (on the other side from the fixed point) the coils you have just made to make another coil.
4. Tighten your knot and slide it along the fixed line to adjust to the tension you desire.

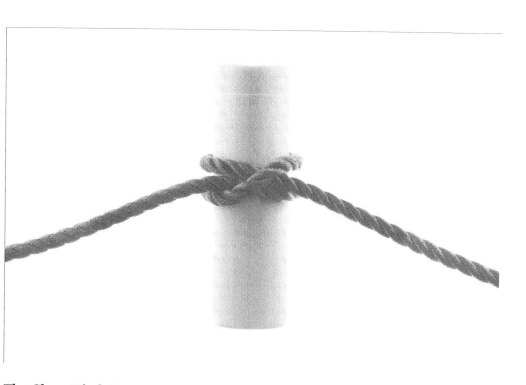

The Clove Hitch Knot

This knot is an easy to learn knot that can be used for securing ropes to trees, poles, or other items that stand verticle. This knot makes it easy to adjust the length of the cord where needed, it is often used when lashing rope-work and also in sailing, especially as a temporary way to hold things.

To make this Knot

1. Wrap the end of your cord, the end that will be loose after you have tied the knot, halfway around the pole or timber you want to anchor your line to.
2. Lay the working end over the wrapped part of the rope to form an X and then wrap it back around the pole.
3. Lift the X shape that you just made in the knot and slip the running end of the cord under the "X" horizontally
4. Pull the knot tight to finish

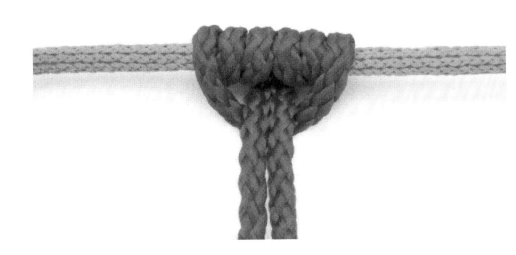

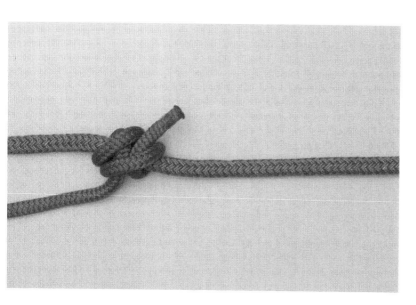

Rolling hitch knot

Rolling hitch knot represents tying a smaller rope to larger rope and stands strongly in the same direction with the standing line. It is mostly used to attach a rope to a post or some other object. If it is tied correctly it will not slip and due to the fact it does not bind it can be tied and untied even with the heavy load on. Sometimes, only when needed, it is recommended to tie one more Rolling hitch knot to the tail end of the first one for security. Rolling hitch is very safe and secure knot to tie. Sailors commonly use the Rolling hitch knot to loosen the pressure on the sheet so it can be cleared of block or a jammed winch.

To make Rolling hitch knot:

1. Take the object and wrap the end of the rope around it.
2. Do it again and go with wrapping it also across the standing line.
3. Wrap it again but this time going above the standing line.
4. Go with the free end under the last wrap and pull firmly to create the knot.

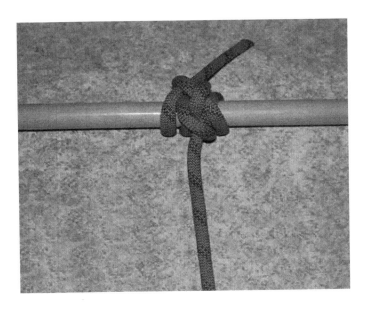

Boom hitch

Boom hitch knot represents safe and very useful knot when you need to attach a rope to a certain object. It can be used when attaching rope to a post, sail boom or securing tent line to a tree branch. It is quite easy to tie requiring only one fold and an Overhand knot.

The Boom hitch is created to bear tension and pulls from either end, but this will largely depend on the finish and the type of rope you use as well.

To make Boom hitch:

1. Start by wrapping turn one around the boom to one side.
2. Wrap turn two around the boom in opposite direction.
3. Turn three needs to be wrapped to original side but going on the top of the first turn.
4. Take turn four and wrapped it both outside and under the turn two.
5. Once you tie an Overhand knot in the tail make sure to tighten it firmly.

The Prusik Knot

A triple sliding hitch knot is also referred to as a Prusik Knot. It is used as a friction hitch knot that's purpose is to apply a loop of cord to a rope so the rope can be used in climbing. It's mainly used in outdoor climbing activities.

To make the Knot

1. Use a cord and make a loop underneath the rope that you want to add the Prusik Knot to.
2. Loop the cord over itself and take over the top of the rope. Pull through the loop. Make sure that the remainder of the cord follows inside of the bight.
3. Repeat the previous step between 3 to 5 times, depending on the thickness of your cord.
4. Bring the cord into the bight once more, but tighten it this time, instead of pulling it completely through.
5. Pull the cord in various directions to add tension to the rope:
6. When you apply a downwards tension it allows the Knot to become and stay tight.
7. When there is no tension the knot will be able to slide loosely up and down the rope

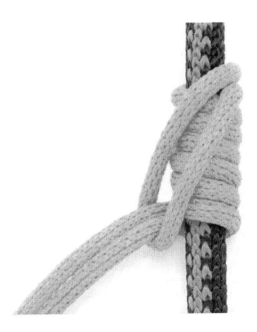

The Klemheist Knot

The Klemheist Knot is tied by making a Prusik Loop with a cord or rope that is no more than 1/2 the diameter of the main, static rope. The friction loop is able to slide up the rope easily, but it will grip the rope when it is subjected to load. The knot will also slide down the rope by pushing the knot without any load on it

To make the Knot

Place a loop consisting of a cord that is no more than 1/2 the diameter of the main line behind the static line.

1. Wrap your line around the static line making the loop on the right side.
2. Repeat step 1, two more times working your way from the bottom to the top.
3. Feed the the loop in the left hand through loop on your right.
4. Pull left loop over to the left side of the static line and pull hard to tighten the knot.
5. Grasp the knot as a whole and slide it up the static line. Secure the knot to the static line with weight to the loop.

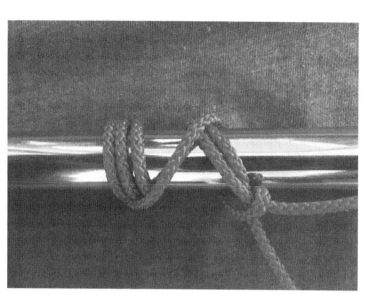

Icicle Hitch knot

The Icicle is quite similar to the Prusik knot and it's best used to connect a line to a post when loaded (i.e. there is weight applied to an end). The difference between Icicle Hitch and other knots is that there is no need for using a loop of rope. Its advantage is that it will hold its place even with a heavy load on a smooth surface. Due to the fact it can hold load both directions makes it excellent knot for climbers. It is a secure knot and very easy to tie.

To make Icicle Hitch knot:

1. Start with twisting the rope around the pole four times in total.
2. Make sure that you're moving away from the pole end.
3. Go with the end of the rope back over the pole against the standing line.
4. Take the hanging loop and pass it behind ends and hook it over the pole.
5. Tie the knot firmly making sure the load is standing against the pole.

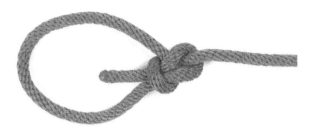

The Bowline

The Bowline is often referred to as "The Rescue knot". This knot creates a loop at the end of your cordage, a loop that cannot shrink or expand. In "The Scouts", this knot is often taught using the story of the rabbit coming out of its hole, in front of the tree, then going behind the tree, and back down his original hole.

The scouts rhyme: Make a loop with the top towards you. The rabbit goes out of the hole, then around the tree, and back into the hole.

How make this Knot

1. Form a loop on top of the long end of the line leaving enough cord for your desired loop size.
2. Just like when you are making an overhand knot, pull the free end of the rope through your loop. Continue around behind the line and then back through the small loop.
3. While maintaining the secondary loop that is going to become your Bowline loop, bring down the free end from the original loop.

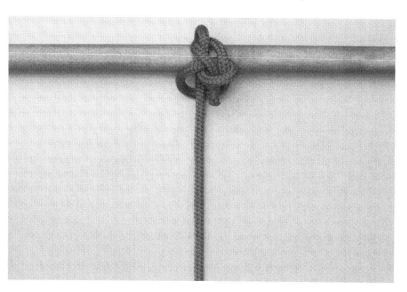

Running Bowline knot

Running Bowline knot is actually a kind of noose, knot or sliding loop that has similarities with the Bowline form in its structure. It is safe and quite strong type of noose that, again, slides easily; it can be simply untied and won't bind.

As the Running Bowline knot is easily undone it has a great purpose in climbing when trying to retrieve objects from places like crevasses, simply by throwing loop that is open around the items and loop itself will tighten around them, as the standing line is pushed very tight. The knot will not bind itself against that standing line which makes it much easier to untie it. It's also used to retrieve overboard rigging and lumber, where Running Bowline knot has found a perfect use.

To make a **Running Bowline knot**:

1. Fold the rope end and wrap the remainder first over, then under the standing line, and to the side of the new loop.
2. By twisting the line you will make a smaller loop on the top of the original loop.
3. Pull the remaining end through the small loop
4. Take that end and wrap it around the top of the large loop and go down through the small one.
5. Tie the end firmly to create the knot through which the main line can slip.

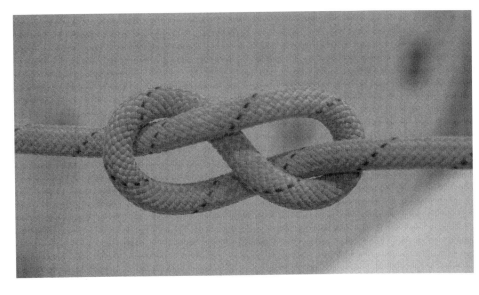

The Figure-Eight Knot

The Figure-Eight Knot is a more secure knot than the most knots; it can be used for preventing cords and ropes from fraying and as a stopper. Rock climbers use it often for tying Caribinas (strong metal snap clips) onto ropes and it is a favorite for securing overhead weights

To make this Knot

1. Tie a single eight in your cord, two feet from its end.
2. Pass the free end through any secure tie-in point if desired.
3. Retrace the original eight with the free end, leaving a loop at the bottom of the size you require.
4. Pull all four strands of cord to cinch down the knot.

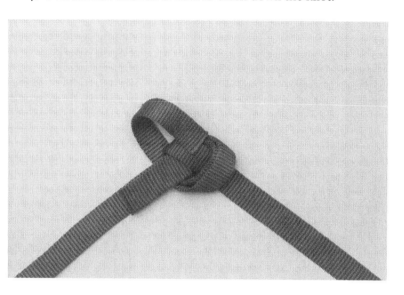

Water (Tape) Knot

Water knot or tape knot can be used to tie two ropes together or to two tape ends. When it's used with the tape it's usually called tape knot. It is mostly used to make sling or a runner.

To make a Water Knot:

1. You need to create an overhand knot – this beginning is same for the tape and for the rope. If you're making a tape knot just bend the tape in the same direction.
2. With the next tape or knot do the same as with the first one, only backward through the knot.
3. When pulling the rope, make sure it goes evenly around the rope or the tape.

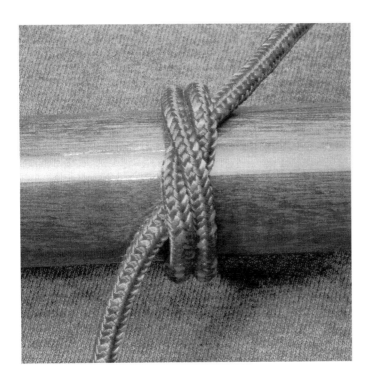

Strangle knot

Strangle knot is basically Binding or Double Overhand knot great for keeping multiple objects together with a rope that goes at least once around the objects, and it can secure the neck of a sack. It is also quite similar to constrictor knot but the main difference between them is that Strangle knot's ends go at the outside edges and with Constrictor knot they go between the turns.

To make a Strangle knot:

1. Go with the rope around the bar and then cross it with the first turn.
2. Pass the rope again going in the same direction.
3. Tuck the rope under the first turns and make sure to tighten them strong enough.

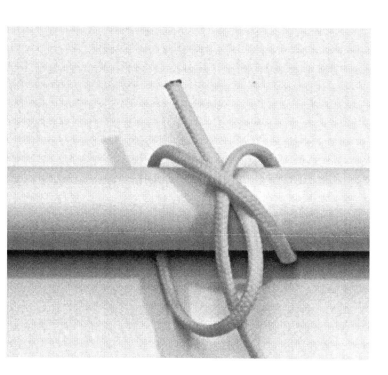

Constrictor knot

Constrictor knot is an excellent binding knot that can keep rope's ends together while being whipped and it can also secure the neck of the sack as well as stick together multiple items. It is probably most effective binding knot. If it is tightened properly it is almost impossible to untightened. Constrictor knot was also used as a clamp. It is also similar to Clove hitch, but when tightened properly it creates an Overhand knot under a riding turn.

To make a Constrictor knot:

1. Pass the rope around the item so its ending goes back over the standing part.
2. Continue wrapping the rope behind the item.
3. Put the ropes working end over the standing part and then pull it underneath both, the riding turn and standing part. That way you'll create an Overhand knot under riding turn.
4. If both ends appear between the turns pull and tight them firmly.

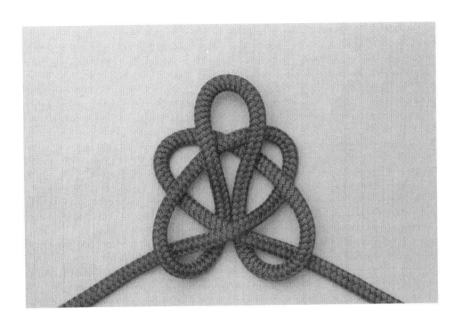

Alpine butterfly loop

The Alpine Butterfly loop is used to create a secure fixed loop in the middle of the rope. Its advantage lies in that that it has possibility to be made in the middle of the rope without having contact with either of the ends which is great for climbers that use long climbing ropes, helping them to isolate damaged parts of rope, creating shorten rope slings and also it comes in handy for climbers that want to hook on a shared rope. It can be safely loaded from multiple directions – in between the two ends where loop hangs freely, from the loop to ends of the rope or load can be spread between both ends. Tying the Alpine butterfly loop you get the possibility to learn more about techniques of tying Alpine Butterfly Bend. Even if it is have loaded Alpine butterfly loop is quite easy to untie.

To make Alpine butterfly loop:

1. Start by wrapping the rope around the hand twice.
2. Place the rope closer to fingertips at the end of the turn one.
3. Make another turn back around your thumb.

4. Take up the turn that is close to your fingertips and make a wrap around the two turns.
5. Take the knot off your hand by sliding it down and firmly tie by pulling the loop and the ends.

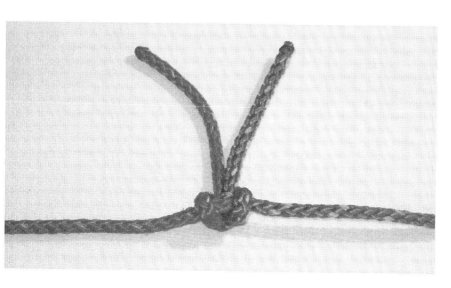

Alpine Butterfly Bend

Alpine butterfly bend is a very reliable and common bend derived from the better-known Alpine Butterfly Loop. It's easy to tie and untie even after being loaded. It's often used by climbers to join two ropes, even if temporarily, and it's very similar to the Zeppelin and the Hunter's loop in that it's interlocking knots overhand. However, its advantage is that it is easily untied with fingers, while the above-mentioned knots would have to be cut to be released.

Besides its strength and reliability, we do believe it's fame also comes from being connected and similar to the Alpine Butterfly Loop – where if you learn one you're half-way through making the other.

To make the Alpine Butterfly bend:

1. Take two ends and join them

2. Wrap the rope around your hand

3. With the joint on the fingertips, go around once more

4. Bend the joint back and under the ropes

5. Slide the knot off your hands and tighten it

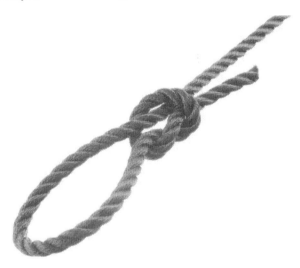

The Slip Knot

The Slip knot is used in various situations. For climbers, Slip knot can be used for tying gear to an anchor or few items attached to it, but it does not secure the anchor itself so it is required to assure that the items are properly attached.

It is very practical due to the fact it can be tied with only one hand and can be made while climbing. The Slip knot is one of the most commonly used knots and it is almost identical to the Noose Knot with the exception that the bight inserted is shaped from the short end and not the long one. It is also used in knitting but only by name as it is almost always structured as noose.

Interestingly, the Slip Knot is sometimes used as temporary stopper knot as well, as it may be used to lock the short end. It's easily untied by pulling one end or tightened around an item if attached to it.

To make the Slip Knot:

1. Fold a loop to double it.
2. Once you have started you can easily decide which end of the rope will actually tighten and which end will untie the Slip Knot.
3. If you are making the Slip knot where you want the right end of the rope to slip, pull the right loop through the left one and if you want the left end to slip you can just send the left loop through the right one.

To be sure it is tightened firmly, straighten it by hand and evenly around the loop.

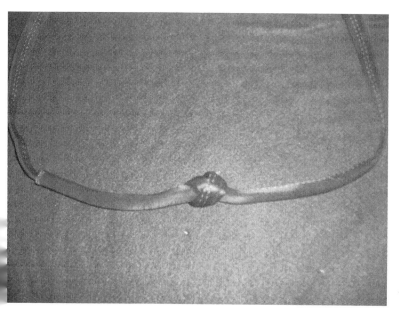

Beer Knot

Beer Knot is used in climbing applications to help climbers create slings or similar devices in rock climbing. It is also used as a loop that joins two parts of tubular webbing together. The Beer Knot knot has more strength, a smaller profile and a much cleaner appearance than the Water knot (which has free-hanging tails). It is much harder to tie the Beer Knot then the Water Knot considering that one of its ends is hidden which makes it as much difficult for safety checks of length tail.

It is wildly known that the Beer Knot is not that easy to slip but it is always good the check out its ends, one is visible and the other is easily felt.

To make Beer Knot:

1. Start by tying an Overhand Knot
2. Make ends and take the pusher rod to hook it on one end.
3. Create the double layer by pulling the rod till his mark.
4. Remove the pusher rod and release the Overhand Knot.
5. Go with the knot around the double layer and tie it strongly.

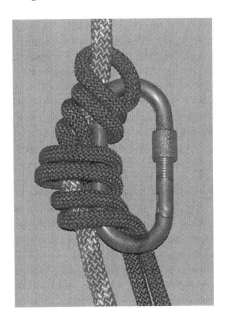

Bachmann knot

The Bachmann knot is actually friction hitch that requires the use of a round cross section carabiner. It is mostly used by arborists or hikers. The knot finds the best use when the friction hitch needs to be constantly or quickly altered, but it's also easily made self-tending so we can say it's multi-practical. The hitch is easily released by grabbing the carabiner while unloading it, sliding and moving up or down when needed.

The best is to use the locking carabiner for Bachmann knot since you will be taking it to move the hitch. Moving the hitch is done by unclipping the top loop and releasing the cord. If you are using a non-locking carabiner, to make sure the knot is safe it is best using it with the gate of carabiner opened facing down. That way it will have much less chance of unclipping itself.

To make Bachmann knot:

1. Make a band of rope or simply use a pre-made tie and put it into the carabiner.
2. Take the strop and wrap it around the rope while holding the carabiner against the rope and then pull the strop through the carabiner.
3. Repeat the action once more if there is a space in the carabiner.
4. Put the load at the bottom of the strop so the knot is in point of friction.

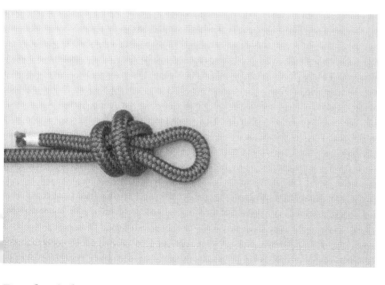

Poacher's knot

Poacher's knot (also known as a variation of Double Overhand knot) is a very secure knot that can be used to create the foot loop to a carabiner or it can be used by cavers in making a cow tail. It is very safe hitch knot. Poacher's knot can be made out of horsehair though it is hard to imagine using that material nowadays.

To make Poacher's knot:

1. Start by creating a bight at the bottom of the rope.
2. Not so tight, wrap its end around that bight two times.
3. Complete the Poacher's knot by pulling its end through those turns.
4. Tighten the knot firmly.

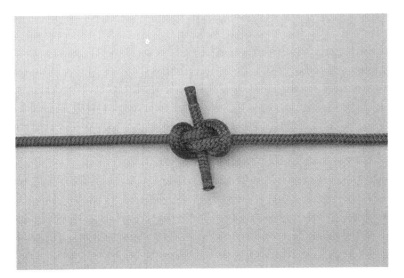

Hunter's bend knot

Hunter's bend knot that is also known as rigger's bend is used to attach two Overhand knots that are the same length. It is quite similar to Zeppelin bend. It is safe and easy to tie and pretty hard to untie when it is heavily loaded. Hunter's bend knot is a great choice when attaching two working ends when knitting. If tied correctly it will never slip.

To make Hunter's bend knot:

1. Take two ropes and create a bight in each of them.
2. Joins those bights together.

3. Go with each end over itself and then over the other rope.
4. Pass the ropes under and across the structure, returning each across and above itself.
5. Make sure to pull firmly creating the finished bend.

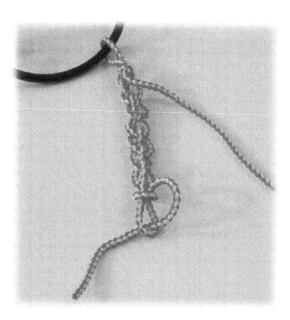

Falconer's knot

Falconer's knot is used in falconry for leashing a bird to a branch. It has a lot of similarities with the Halter hitch knot with the exception that you can tie Falconer's knot with only one hand while holding the bird with your other hand. To be able to hold the bird it is better to use stiff leash instead of the flexible.

To make Falconer's knot:

1. Take the rope and go with it around the glove with the tail end on the left side.
2. Holding both parts of the rope, lock the tail in between your first and middle finger.
3. Put your thumb on the two pieces, under the second and then take it to the right.

4. Turn your wrist right so that back of the hand is facing up and your thumb should create the loop.
5. Go with the rope through the loop
6. Pull the free end through this loop and tie it strongly.

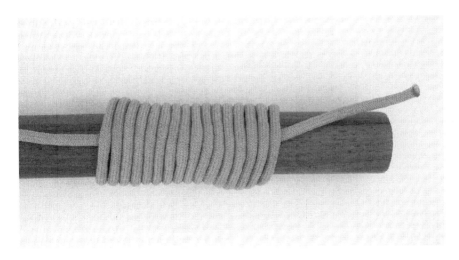

The Common Whipping

The Common Whipping knot is typical whipping knot or number of knots tied at the bottom of the rope to prevent the end from loosening and its advantage is that it can be tied without using the needle or any other tool. The Common Whipping knot is very easily tied and also very secure with no visible ends if correctly tied. Its disadvantage is that it can slide very easily of the end of the rope if any of the turns get cut. Since it can slide, it is best to use this knot with natural fiber rope and natural twine then the synthetic one, because it will hold it at the end of the rope and prevent from unraveling. Again, if used with synthetic rope it is best to wrap it with the tape to avoid the slipping.

To make a Common Whipping Knot:

1. Put the twine along the rope.
2. Create a bight back on the rope.
3. The rope is supposed to be whipped near its end.
4. Firmly wrap the twine around the rope and the bight of twine.

5. Continue wrapping until the whipping is at least double as wide as the rope itself.
6. Wrap the working end of the twine through the bight.
7. By slowly pulling the standing end of the twine you will get both the bight and working end to go under the whipping.
8. Trim the ends to complete the knot.

Chapter 3: Sailing Knots

The ropes used in marine conditions, especially boating are usually very durable and expensive as most boat owners only use high quality cords or ropes with the emphasis on safety, reliability and convenience rather than the cost, as these ropes are used repeatedly. As a rule, all of the ropes used in boats need to be able to handle extreme conditions and heavy loading such as is found when berthing, mooring, towing, tying down for storm preparation or sail and rigging work. The types of knots used have to be capable of doing the job required as often lives and property depend on their integrity and ease of application, both to tie and untie each knot without difficulty especially in adverse weather conditions.

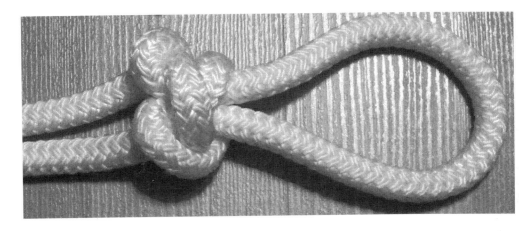

The Lineman's Loop

The lineman's loop is a knot used to form a loop in the middle of a ropeor cord when you do not have access to the ends. This knot will handle significant amounts of weight on the loop and the ends and it is also good withloading from all directions. The shape of this loop makes it easy in the case that you need to inspect it.

To make the Knot

1. First, make a large bight (loop) in the area of the cord you want to have the finished loop

2. Twist the bight to form 2 loops, a large loop on top with a smaller one under it.

3. Fold the top loop over the bottom loop so that smaller, bottom loop is inside the larger loop

4. Take the farthest edge of the bottom loop from the first loop and bring that through the second (smaller) loop.

5. Tighten the knot, allowing the ends to tighten themselves while you tighten the whole knot.

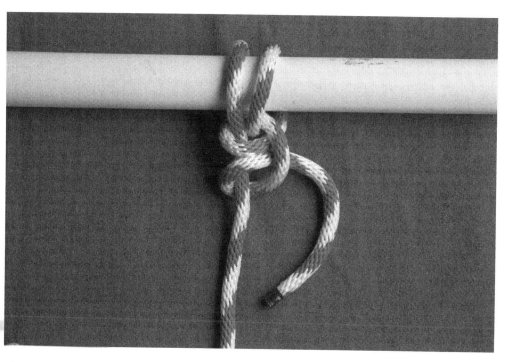

The Anchor Hitch

The Anchor hitch or fisherman's hitch as would be expected from its name, is an excellent knot for attaching an anchor line to a chain or anchor eye.

To make the Knot

1. First pass the cord through the anchor ring from behind it.
2. Then pass it through the anchor ring once more in the same direction.
3. Continue feeding the cord under the standing part and through the 2 loops.
4. Then pass it under the standing part, then over it and through the loop, making a half hitch.
5. Make a second half hitch and then seize the tail end to the line (Tie it off with twine)

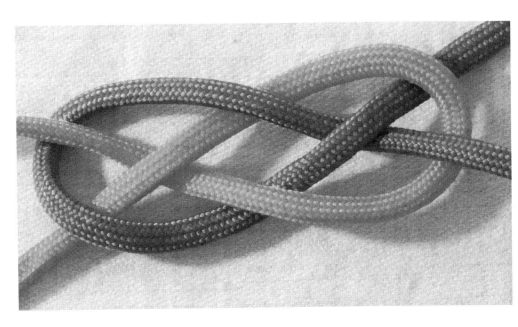

The Carrick Bend

The Carrick bend is also known as a Sailors Hitch and Josephine knot, it is a basic knot that is often used to join a short cord or cable to a longer one. It is particularly suited to using with cords or rope that is too thick or stiff for many other types of knots, it gives an excellent grip under all conditions including wet, oily and slippery conditions. It is also easy to untie, even under load.

To make this Knot

If you are using one cord,

1. Make a bight (loop) in the cord.
2. Take the shorter end and loop it over the long end, pulling it up straight.
3. Slide the short end down, below where the cord originally crossed to form your first loop, and then tighten both ends of the cord.

If you are using two cords and wish to join them together

1. First, start by making a bight (loop) with the first rope.
2. Place a second cord directly over the first one, looping it under the long end of the first cord, but over the short end.
3. Form another loop with the second cord
4. Take the end you used in step 3 and bring it back over the longer end, causing it to intersect over the second cord and over itself, and then finish it under the short end.
5. Tighten the knot by applying tension to all four ends of the cords equally.

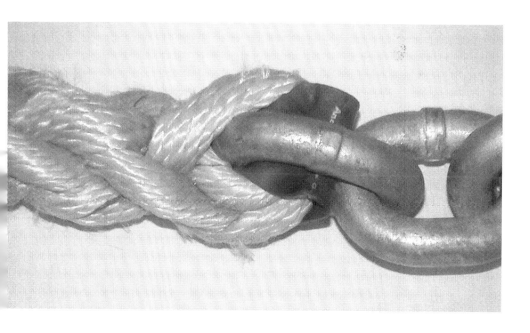

The Chain Splice

Splicing a rope or cord to a chain is usually done when a chain and cord combination has to pass over a windlass and then go down into a chain locker.

To make the Splice (knot)

1. Undo the braid on the cord or rope and divide these strands into 3 equal sized strands, it is usual to undo a measured 21 times the cord's diameter and then wrap the rope at this point with tape or twine to stop it unraveling further.
2. Push 2 strands together through the end of the chain up to the point where you tied the main cord off
3. Then pass a 3rd strand through in the reverse direction
4. Lay the 3 strands down beside the cord and thread them into the cord using a spike to open the weave, starting as close to the chain as possible
5. Complete the splice by tucking the rest of the strands into the cord in line with the existing weave or pattern. Once the first 3 tucks are made, it is necessary to remove the twine so that the splice can be pulled tight up against the chain or anchor eye.

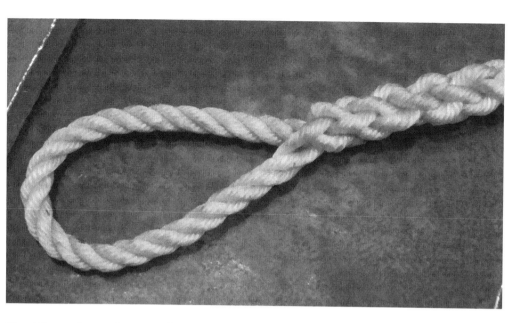

The Three Strand Eye Splice

This eye splice is made or used when you require a permanent soft eyed loop or eye at the end of a cord for attaching or joining to other applications.

To make the Knot (splice)

1. Most cords or ropes are made up of many strands that usually stay together because of the twist of the cord or rope. Separate the strands into 3 equal parts by unraveling or separating the cord, the usual length needed is at least the amount of cord needed to wrap around the cord 5 times (a little extra can easily be trimmed off at the end).
2. Seal the ends of the strands to prevent them unraveling while you work and place a few rounds of tape (insulation tape works well) on the ends of each strand to stiffen them and make it easier to work and pass through the weave of the cord.
3. Place a round of tape or twine at the point of the cord where you stopped separating the strands to stop it unraveling further.
4. Determine the size of loop or eye you require

5. Loosen the base of your loop and feed in your first strand. Usually you will be able to untwist the cord, but sometimes a spike or a small screwdriver may be needed to break them apart.
6. Keep the strands separated and feed the first one into the main body of the rope as close to the tape as possible, try and follow the pattern or weave of the strands there with each strand you feed into the loosened main part of the cord, so it will look and feel right.
7. Tuck your second strand end into the weave pattern so that it passes under the strand at the base of your loop and up through the space between the strands. Then pull it through so it emerges, going through and out of the space between the strands in the cord.
8. Tuck your last strand end into the weave; it should be obvious where it goes if you are watching the pattern develop.
9. Draw the ends tight using both of your hands to pull the end strands through the loose strands at the bottom of the loop. Repeat this until the end of the rope at the bottom of the end strand joins the loose strand at the bottom of your loop and all of the strands are tight.
10. Continue the weave of the splice by loosening the weave of the main body of your cord as you go and tucking the strands in following the strand pattern of the main cord. For most types of rope you will need to make 5 tucks of each strand into the main cord to ensure that the splice does not slip. This is because almost all modern synthetic cords or ropes are by nature slippery, so need an extra safety margin.

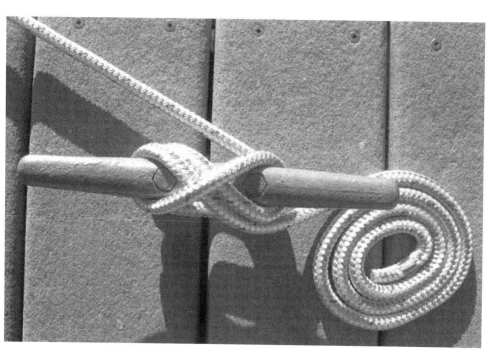

The Cleat Hitch

The Cleat Hitch or knot is deceptively simple, yet it is often made the wrong ay by the inexperienced, if it is not done correctly, it can be impossible to undo when under load.

To make this Knot

1. At the start the cord or rope must feed around the most distant horn of the cleat followed by a turn in the same direction around the other horn.
2. After passing the cord around the 2 horns of the cleat, the cord must cross over to form the figure 8 turns. The number of turns is dependent on the size of the cleat and the size of the cord or rope. It is recommended that a cleat hitch should never be finished with a half hitch, but it is acceptable to make a half hitch in the line a little way up from the cleat to keep it from cluttering the deck, as long as it can be reached easily and quickly.
3. The modern synthetic ropes that most people use are stronger, thinner, more slippery and more elastic than traditional ropes (a nylon rope will stretch more

than 5% when loaded to 20% of its rated breaking load) so this should be taken into account.

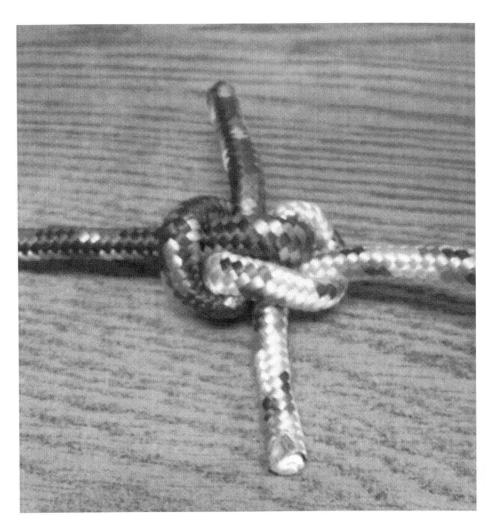

The Zeppelin Bend

The Zeppelin knot is one of the strongest, most secure knots commonly used, although it may look complicated, if you go slowly and follow instructions, it's can be easy and actually quite simple.

Basically to make this knot you make two loops and joining them together, forming one single knot. It is always important to test any knot including the zeppelin, before placing a load on it to assure it is secure before using it in any situation and especially if they are used where their failure could jeopardize people or property.

If working with heavy, tough or stiff cords, it may be difficult to maneuver them, so to make working them easier, using both hands or asking a friend to assist you to hold the rope in place as you make the loops may be necessary.

To make this knot

1. To start, first check your cord for any tangles or knots. Make sure that the rope is free of any obstructions.
2. Place two pieces of cord on a flat surface, forming a straight line with a small break in between the line.
3. With the left hand cord form a counterclockwise loop, it is important to place the tail of the left rope over the rest of the rope, forming a q-like shape. Do not place it under the rest of the rope
4. With the right hand cord form a clockwise loop, this is basically the opposite of what you did with the left hand cord. Pass the end of the right cord under the remaining cord. For the knot to tie or work correctly the loops must be perfect mirror images of each other, with one tail hanging over the remaining rope, while the other rope should have the tail passing under.
5. Place the left loop on top of the right loop so that the loop with the tail is on top of the excess cord that goes on top of the loop with the tail end on the bottom of the remaining rope.
6. If necessary get assistance to keep the cords in place while you work.
7. Take the tail of the left loop and pass it through the two stacked loops of rope, ensuring that the tail end of the left loop passes under the circle formed by the two ropes. Do not pass the tail end of the left rope over the circle·
8. Then do the same with the right loop's tail, Take the tail of the right loop through the two loops of cord, the circle, passing the tail end on top the stacked loops.

9. To finish the knot, pull on the long ends until the knot is tight and secure, not the tail ends of the two ropes. Pulling on the tail ends will undo the knot so you will have to start again.

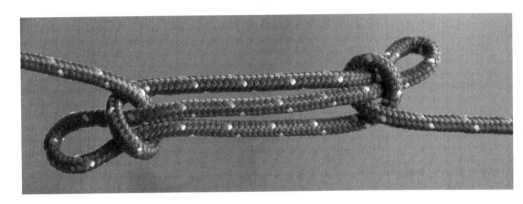

The Sheepshank Knot

The sheepshank is mainly used for one of two purposes, either as a means to shorten a rope without cutting it, this can be handy when both ends are secure and you can not get to them, the other use is to by-pass a damaged section of a cord or rope without having to cut it (the damaged part would be in the center, where there is no tension).

The main disadvantage is this knot can undo if there is no tension on it, so to use it safely it needs tension applied on both sides of the knot at all times. It is also best suited to using with a coarse or rough rope, not a synthetic rope as it could fail when it becomes slippery even under tension. Often when this knot is used a separate cord is tied through the loops at each end of the finished knot, to form a safeguard in case of a failure.

To make the Knot

1. First, make an "S" shape in the cord that incorporates the area you wish to shorten the cord by. The "S" shape is really 2 bights loops).

2. The center part will have no tension on it.
3. Form loops on the ends of the 2 bights
4. Put the two bights into the loops and then pull the loose ends tightly to tighten the knot.

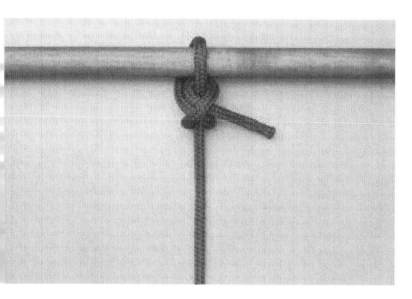

Buntline Hitch

The Buntline hitch has been used by sailors to tie a rope to an item, popular for its simplicity and effectiveness. It's very secure as shaking and pulling further stiffen and tighten the hitch rather than untie or loosen it. The Buntline hitch will jam when loaded to the extreme so it's often formed in slipped form, with materials such as Dyneema Hollow Braid.

To make a Buntline Hitch:

1. Pull the rope around a pole or stick.
2. Make sure to make a full turn around the standing end and through the hoop closer to the pole.
3. Pass the rope around and under itself once more to complete the knot (which is actually forming a simple half hitch).

You can pass a bight through instead of the end if you'd like to make a slipped form, where you'd easily release the hitch by pulling the bight back.

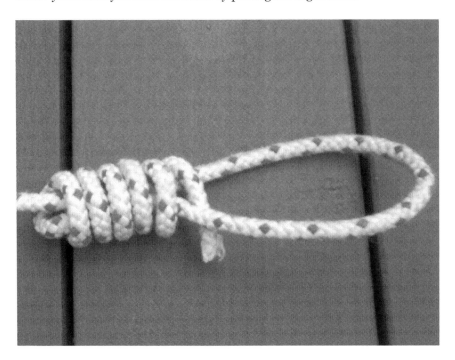

Heaving Line Knot

There are many knots that can be considered a heaving line knot family, where we actually add weight at the end of the rope to it can be thrown more easily. We create a simple, heavy knot often used in sailing and climbing, often attached to the main rope and impossible to remove. It's important to note that there are other more complicated and distinct knots sharing the name, usually adding specific details to it.

To make a simple Heaving Line knot:

1. Create a bight and grip it so to circle the tail end.
2. Wrap the end taking just two strands once.
3. Then wrap the whole structure (all three strands) until you use up the tail end of the rope.
4. Pull it through the loop made.

5. Finish by tightening the knot, by pulling the end loop and the standing end.

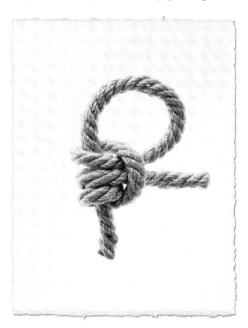

Lighterman's Hitch

The Lighterman's Hitch (also known as Tugboat Hitch) is a simple knot often used in towing, being very easy to make, loaded and released even under heavy weight. There is no actual knot about it, it takes the heavy load with a rope passed around the standing end in two directions, putting a bight over post each time the direction is changed.

While it's very simple and easy to untie, it's important to take extreme care when tying as it can cause issues loosening if not tied tightly to start with. When untying, the tail gets a very good use as to control the load after each turn.

To make a Lighterman's Hitch:

1. Wrap the rope around a post twice.
2. Put a bight on the post but under the standing end.
3. Wrap another turn, then put another bight the same way.

4. This will take the initial tension and provide control over the weight until you complete the hitch.

5. Complete the hitch by adding as many turns as you may need.

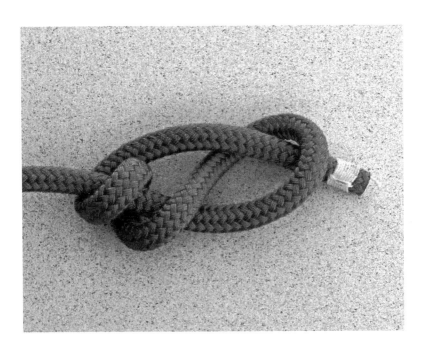

Stevedore knot

As its name says - it was named after stevedores – people in charge to load and unload the ship goods. Stevedore knot was mainly used as the stopper while unloading cargo and it was usually tied near the end of the rope to prevent unreeving. To be able to raise and lower the cargo, stevedores used blocks which required the need to use larger stopper knot that will secure that the line does not go straight through the block.

It is a rater bulky knot which makes it a perfect stopper knot. Stevedore knot is very easy to tie and also easy to untie even with the heavy loading.

To make Stevedore knot:

1. Start by making a bight at the bottom of the rope.

2. Go over the standing line with the working end and continue until you make a full round.
3. Repeat this action two or three more times making full rounds around standing line going back to the bottom of the rope.
4. Once you pull the end through the bight, tie down the turns.
5. Take both ends and tie them strongly creating the Stevedore knot

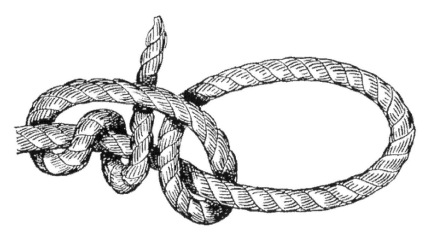

Midshipman's Hitch

Midshipman's Hitch is a great choice and a better alternative of the somewhat better known Tautline knot, as it is more secure and has an Awning Hitch which takes any tension while making the Half Hitch. The Midshipman's hitch allows creating a modifiable loop at the end of a rope, which can then be skidded up and down routinely changing the size of the loop and the length of the line.

It's also easy to tie and release under load, even under extreme weight which is another advantage, especially for boating purposes.

To make a Midshipman's Hitch:

1. Wrap the tail end around standing end twice.
2. Pass the end through the first turn and pull tight (creating the Awning Hitch).
3. Go around and make a half hitch (creating the Midshipman's Hitch).

4. Finally, if you'd like to make it Adjustable, you can easily do it by making a half hitch in reverse.

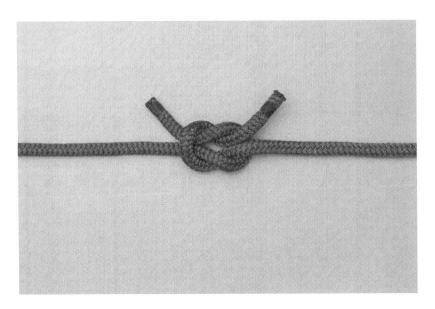

Square Knot

The Square Knot is also known as Reef Knot due to the fact it was used through the history by sailors for reefing sails. It is great for securing items that are not critical. It is very easy to tie the Square Knot but it is not safe to tie two ropes together because it can easily be untied so it shouldn't be used as a bend. His safety is not very high but it can be used for many other purposes like tying sail over the sail or it can tie the string on a gift. Learning how to tie Square Knot gives you an insight in technics of tying Half Hitch Knot or Half Knot.

To make Square Knot:

1. Start by crossing two ropes to create a half knot.
2. First cross the left over right and then the right over left.
3. Take their ends and tie them firmly into Square Knot

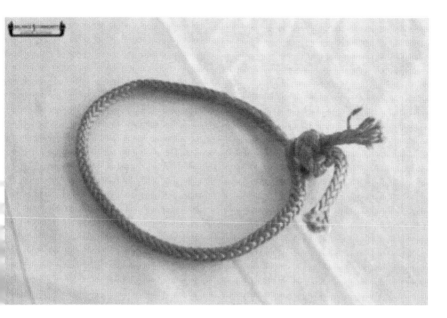

Soft Shackle

Soft shackles are a great replacement for metal shackles in yachting, as they're a lot cheaper and safer variant for the crew members. They will also not wear out the casting and/or rails, while there is next to no chance of it getting undone when secured. Soft shackles are widely recommended as a better alternative in almost all conditions, except when having to undo under load or bringing ends together very tightly before securing them.

To make a Soft Shackle:

1. Measure the rope and highlight where you'll enter and exit the rope with a fid.
2. Slide the fid in and form an eye at the top, getting two ends on the lower end.
3. Slide the fid through the inner rope so that you can now pull the outer rope through it.
4. Pull both ends to make them equal in length.
5. Make a Lanyard Knot with the two ends.
6. Pull a part of the rope through the eye to make a small loop.
7. Take the Lanyard Knot through it.

8. Tighten the shackle as needed.

It's important to note there are variations, where Edwards' soft shackle (considered the best, but not the most elegant soft shackle) has two parallel lines for a short, while Kohlhoff Shackle has the two lines running all the way around.

Chapter 4: Necktie Knots

Not all ties are tied in the same way, in fact, there are many variations or ways to tie a necktie, just as all ties are not the same, knots can vary in size, symmetry and shape, every knot has its own distinct character that is suitable for different types or styles of necktie. When deciding on the type of knot to use consideration should be made for the thickness, width and length of the tie as well as the style of shirt and collar and your desired look. Often a thick tie necessitates the use of a smaller type knot such as the Four in Hand, while thin ties usually look better with larger style knots such as the Windsor or Pratt. The following are a few of the most popular ways to tie a tie.

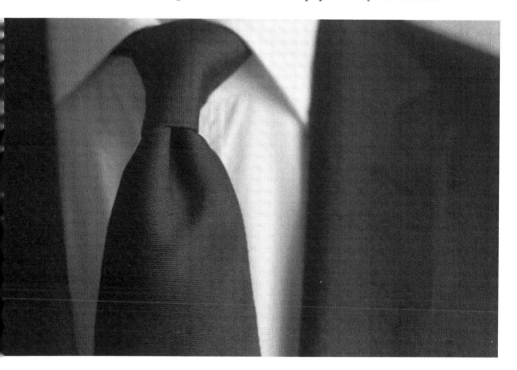

Four In Hand Knot

This knot is a style that can be used for button-down shirts, it works well with wider ties that are made from heavier materials. The four in hand knot is mainly a technique for beginners or for, novices, although it can be easily learned by people who just want a new style or way to tie their necktie.

To tie the Four in Hand Knot

1. Place your tie around your neck and below your shirt collar, with the wider portion of your tie on the right side and the thinner portion on the left side.
2. Adjust the lengths so that the end of the wide side is 12 to 15 inches (30 to 38 cm) lower than the thinner portion.
3. First, cross the wider portion of the tie over the thinner portion to the left and hold the 2 sides of the tie together in that position with your right hand.
4. Then change hands so that your left hand is holding the tie in position at the intersection of the tie.
5. Take the wide portion back below the narrow portion from left to right.
6. Then, switch to hold the intersection of the two ends with your left hand and turn the wider portion back below the thinner portion from left to right.
7. Now bring the wider portion of the tie back over to the left in front of the thinner portion using your right hand.
8. Then, bring the wider portion under the knot and pull this wider portion up and through the loop
9. Now take the wider portion of the tie and pass through the front of the knot.
10. Pull down gently on the thinner portion of the tie with one hand, and slowly move the knot up to the center of the collar with the other hand.
11. The wider portion of the tie should just reach the top of your belt buckle (that is assuming you are wearing standard not low slung pants).

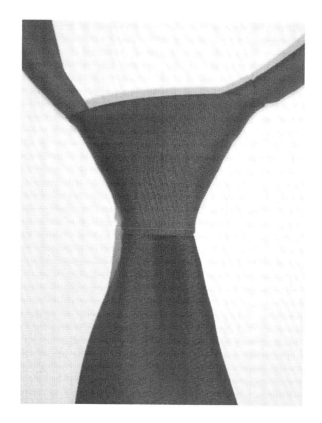

The Half Windsor

The half Windsor is the style tie tying that most men prefer, this is because it is considered to be more distinguished than the four in hand knot and it is not as bulky as the full Windsor.

To make the Half Windsor Knot

1. It helps to start tying this knot while looking in a mirror, so you can see what you're doing. Place the tie around your neck with the wider portion draped down about 10 or 12 inches (25 or 30 cm) below the thin end to start with.
2. First loop the wider portion around the thinner portion. Then bring the wider portion over the thinner portion, and then behind it, creating a loop.
3. Lift the wider portion out in front of your body, then flip it over and tuck it into the space between the tie and your collar.

4. Then bring the wider portion out to the front, and cross it over the thinner portion from right to left.

5. Tuck the wider portion up through the loop by bringing it up between the loop and collar.

6. Then pull the wider portion through the knot in the front of the tie. Tighten and adjust so that the knot has an even shape.

7. To finish tightening the tie around your collar, pull on the narrow side of the tie, which should now be hidden below the wide side of the tie. If your tie has a carrier loop below the wider portion of the tie, you may slide the smaller side through the loop to keep it from showing from behind the wider part of the tie.

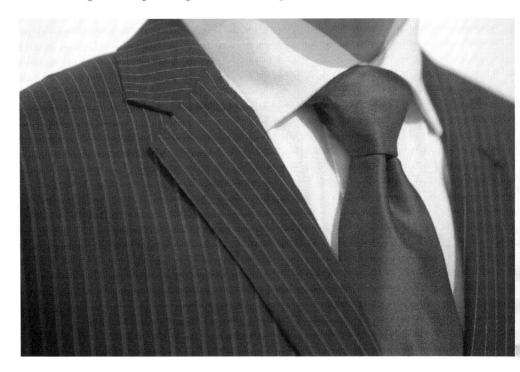

The Windsor Knot

The Windsor knot is considered by many to be the most elegant way to tie a tie, it is most suitable for the wide spread type of shirt collar.

To tie the Windsor Knot

1. Start by standing in front of a mirror, if you are looking at what you're doing in the mirror, it will make it much easier to tie this knot. Check that your shirt is buttoned to the top and stand your collar up before proceeding.

2. Place your tie around your neck, normally one end of the tie will be considerably wider than the other. If you are left handed, switch the sides of the wide and narrow side and reverse the following instructions as you go!

3. Cross the wide side of the tie over the thin side to make an X the thinner side will or should then be located on the bottom and the wider side on top.

4. There should be a V that was created from the X that you made and the collar of the shirt,this should a form a loop. Intersect the wide portion of your tie below the thin portion and pull it through the loop.

5. Bring the wider portion of the tie back down to where it was before you looped it through the upper V.

6. Then pull the wider portion of the tie below the thinner portion and to the right, then back through the "V" loop and to the right again, so that the wider portion is inside out.

7. Cross the wide portion over the thin portion again, going to the right.

8. Then cross the wider portion over the thinner portion, creating an "X" shape again with the thinner side, located on the bottom and the wider side on top. This will form a loose knot around the thinner end.

9. Take the wider portion that you just pulled through the loop and put it through the loose knot and pull it all the way through.

10. Tighten until the knot is about an inch below the collar.

11. Fold down your collar, and adjustment to make sure that the knot is placed directly in the center of the collar.

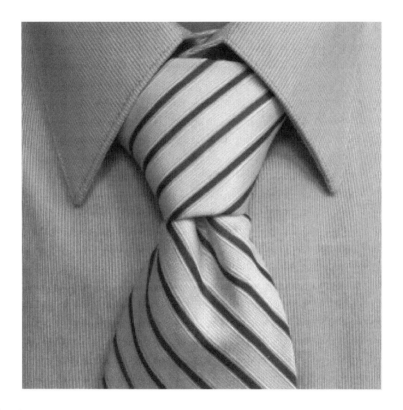

Pratt Knot

If you are searching for a bigger knot that looks classy with a wide collar dress shirt, then mastering the Pratt or Shelby is probably the style for you. It looks good with any dress shirt and wider neckties that are made out of lighter fabrics.

To make the Knot

1. The Pratt is one of the few knots that start with the necktie inside out.
2. Start with the wider portion on the right, letting it extend about 12 inches (30cm) below the thinner portion on the left and then cross the wider portion under the thinner portion.
3. Take the wide portion over and under the thinner end. Pulling the loop down to tighten.
4. Next, pull the wider portion over to the right.
5. Pull the wider portion up, behind the loop.

6. Take the wider portion of the tie and pull it down through the loop in front of the tie.
7. Tighten gently while firmly holding both sides.

Prince Albert Knot

The Prince Albert knot is a variation on the Victoria knot, named after Prince Albert, husband of Queen Victoria. In the Prince Albert knot the wide or active end is passed through both the first and second turnings. This knot is a little bit more bulky but it can be pulled tight to give it a different look.

To make the Knot

1. Place the tie around your neck with the wider portion of the tie on the right side and the thinner portion on the left.
2. Only move the active (wide) end.
3. Place the wider portion over the thinner portion to the left.
4. Then, under the small end and to the right.
5. Then, across the front and to the left.
6. Then, under the small end and to the right.
7. Then across the front and to the left.
8. Now, up through the neck loop from below.
9. And finally through both loops in the front.
10. Tighten your knot by pulling on the wider portion. Slide the knot up & adjust.
11. The first loop should show slightly below the second loop.

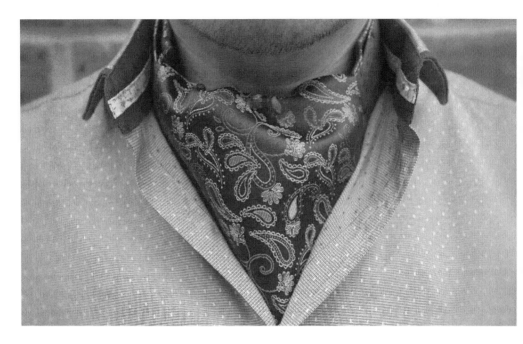

The Cravat or Ascot

The ascot became popular with the psychedelic music in the late 1960s and again in the 1970s. The main differences between a tie and a cravat are that a cravat is usually shorter, wider and of softer material than a tie and is worn against the skin whereas a tie is placed under the collar on the shirt.

To make the Cravat or Ascot Knot

1. Place the cravat around your neck, inside your collar with the two open ends resting on your chest.
2. Some cravats have a loop already sewn onto one side, if the one you have has this feature, simply pull the long portion of the cravat through that preexisting loop and move on to step 5
3. Pull one end of your cravat about six inches lower than the other.
4. Then cross the long end over and in front of the short end.
5. If you want the knot to be tighter and more secure knot, wrap the long end around the short end a second time.

6. Tuck the long end up and under the short end at the base of the neck. Do not make the folds too tight.
7. Pull the long end of the cravat all the way through and straighten it out.
8. Adjust the cravat so that the long end is directly on top of the short end in the center of your chest just like a normal tie with the two ends about the same length.
9. The part of the cravat that should be visible is the bib that forms around the neck, the rest is usually tucked into a vest waistcoat or placed under the 2nd button of a shirt.

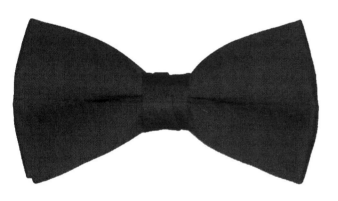

Bowtie knot

Bow tie knot is used to tie bow tie mostly for elegant occasions like weddings or typical events that are perfect opportunities to wear the bow tie and to give you a formal appearance.

To make a Bowtie knot:

1. Place your Bowtie under your collar and around the neck. One part should be just a bit longer than the other.
2. Take the longer part and cross it with the shorter one.
3. Create a half knot and keep it tight with your finger
4. Band shorter part in half and then put the longer part over it.
5. The part that is unfolded band into half fold.
6. Push the bow tie through the loop behind the bow but only half way.
7. Take the bow tie by the ends and pull thigh so it's even on both sides and make sure it is at the middle of the collar.

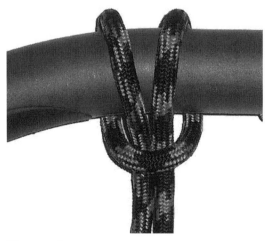

Hoxton knot

Hoxton knot is actually a way of tying the scarf around the neck and it is also known as Chelsea knot, Snug Tug or French loop. It is quite popular among celebrities such as football players or TV shows hosts.

To make a Hoxton knot:

1. Take scarf, fold it, and then place it around your neck
2. The both ends of the scarf need to go through the folded part.
3. Tighten slightly.

Chapter 5: Fisherman's Knots

Knots used for fishing lines are slightly different than knots used in most other applications because they are generally designed to be tied using monofilament or braided fishing line. These knots have to be able to run through the eyes and rungs of fishing rods and other types of rigs. They are usually not designed to be untied because fishing line is very cheap and the knots have to be very tight with multiple tightly wound turns, making untying difficult, this means these knots are usually cut off rather than being untied. These knots are also designed to avoid as much as possible the loss of line strength caused by the knots. Controlled testing shows that monofilament with a knot in its length will break at about 50% of its ideal strength, a well made and designed knot will reduce the chances of knot failure and line breakages.

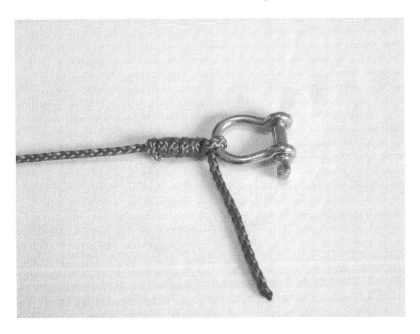

Clinch Knot

The clinch knot is one of the most widely used knots of commercial and sports fishermen. It provides an excellent method of securing the main line to a hook, lure or swivel with fishing lines that are under 30 lb test load.

To make this Knot

1. First pass the end of your line through the eye, leaving enough line to work, about 6in to 1 ft.
2. Wrap the line around the standing end or eye about 5 complete turns.
3. Pass the end back through the loop beside the eye.
4. Then pass the end under the final turn.
5. Wet the knot to lubricate it, and then tighten it and trim off any excess.

The Non- Slip Mono Knot

The non-slip Mono Knot or Lefty Kreh's Loop Knot as it is also known as, is a high strength fixed loop in the end of a line knot that doesn't grip the lure allowing for a flexible attachment which has the effect of providing a more natural action on the lure.

To make this Knot

1. Loosely tie an overhand knot in your line about 6 inches from the end.
2. Pull the tag end of the line through the opening of your lure or swivel and then pass it reversely into the opening of the overhand knot.
3. Then pull the tag end of the line around the fixed end, approximately five or six times and then pass it back through the overhead knot.
4. Wet the knot with water or vegetable oil to lubricate it and then tighten it, trim the end close to the knot

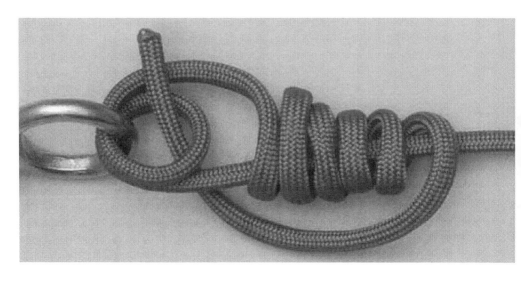

TRILENE KNOT

The Trilene Knot is a stronger version of the Clinch knot, it has been shown in tests to retain a much higher percent of the line's original strength. It is especially easy to tie with lighter fishing lines of under 30 lbs.

To make the Knot.

1. Start by running about 6 to 8 inches of line through the hook eye or swivel, then run it through again forming a small loop.
2. Run your tag end of the tie through the eye two times, making a small loop.
3. Hold the loop firmly, then bring the tag end of the line around the standing line at least five times and then pass the end back through the loop
4. Moisten the knot thoroughly with water or vegetable oil and then tighten the knot

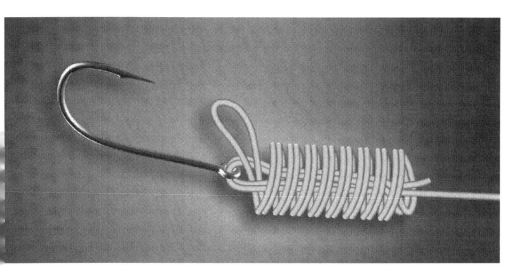

The Berkley Braid Knot

The Berkley Braid Knot has been reported to be a good choice that works well with all fishing lines as well as braided fishing lines. It is said it has few weaknesses and is simple to make or apply.

To make the Knot

1. To start, double the main line into a bight (loop).
2. Pass the doubled line / bight through the eye of the hook and then back up the main line.
3. Wrap the line around the main line and the loop line, making 8 wraps around it starting at the top going down towards the eye.
4. Thread the end of the loop into the hole between the eye and last wrap.
5. Lubricate the knot using water or vegetable oil, then tighten it by pulling on the main rope, tag end and loop
6. Trim the tag end and the loop

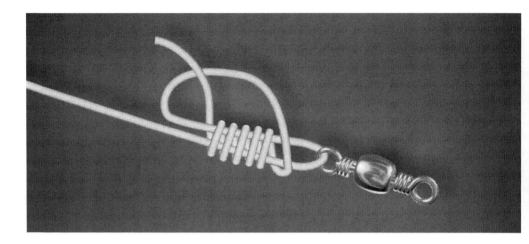

UNI-TO-UNI KNOT

When you need to join fishing lines (or any other type of line, cord or rope) of relatively similar diameters, the Uni to Uni Knot has been shown to give consistently good results The Uni to Uni preserves up to 90 percent of line strength, and is a stronger connection than many of the other popular knots. If making the knot using cords or lines that are of different diameters, add several more turns to the thin line to remove any chance of it slipping or if failing.

To make the Knot

1. Place the lies to be joined end to end with at least 6 to 8 inches of overlap.
2. Take the end of one of the lines and fold it back to the halfway mark of the overlapped lines forming a bight or loop to the halfway point.
3. Make 6 to 8 wraps around both of the lines towards the loop and pass the end through that loop.
4. Pull tag end of the same line to tighten it.
5. Repeat the process in the other line, making 6 to 8 wraps around both of the lines towards the loop and pass the end through that loop.
6. Pull tag end of the same line to tighten it.
7. Lubricate the knot with water or vegetable oil and pull both lines in opposite directions to slide the two knots together and finish the knot.

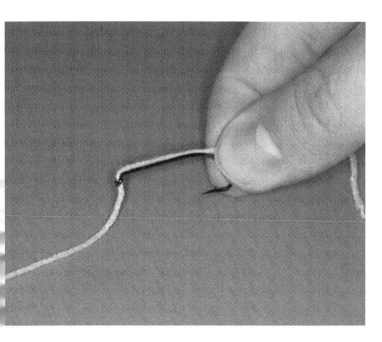

Knotless knot

One of the most popular knots among fisherman is definitely the Knotless knot. When tied properly, attaching the fishing hook to the fishing line, it leaves the space for various baits in the loop section. The loop section is actually certain length of line left to hang below the hook and it is also known as "hair rig".

To make Knotless knot:

1. To be able to hold the bait, the loop needs to be tied at the end of the line.
2. The other end needs to be pulled through the eye of the hook and then adjust the loop to wanted position and length.
3. Go double back and create 5 – 8 wraps around the hook shank making those turns as neat as possible.
4. Once you finish wraps, pull the free end through the eye of the hook.
5. Holding the loop end, pull the free end firmly and wrap up to the eyed hook.
6. Make sure to use a drop of rig glue on the knot.

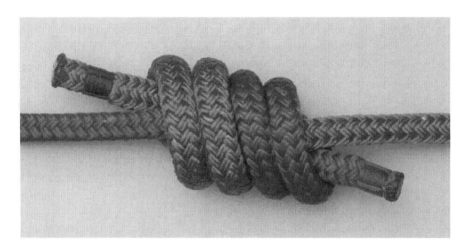

Double fisherman knot

Double fisherman knot is very reliable and it is an excellent knot that can join two ropes together or their ends creating a safe loop. It is also known as Grapevine knot and it is used in many situations like search and rescue or climbing. It is also used in fishing, although not that often, creating the finishing knot with two tightened knots that slide together.

Kayakers and rafters often use the Double fisherman knot to make the so-called "grab handles" for their boats, tying it in short lengths of rope on each end of the boat. This knot is created by making a Double overhand knot but represented in its Strangle knot form.

To make a Double fisherman knot:

1. Take two ends and overlap them.
2. One end of the rope wrap two times around the other rope and pull it back through the inside of the coils tying it firmly.
3. Do the same with the other rope but only in the opposite direction.
4. Pull the ends to strongly tie the knots making them slide together.

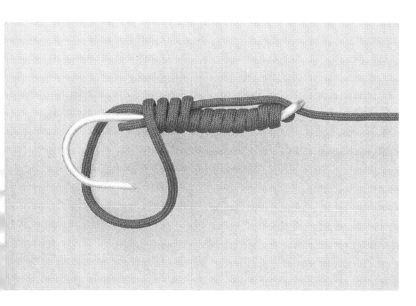

Egg Loop knot

Egg Loop knot is mostly used by fishermen and it's very practical, especially when fishing for Salmon or Steelhead. It provides a loose bait using clusters of eggs attached to a hook. It is also called Bait loop or Bumper loop. Most important thing to care about when tying the Egg Loop knot is to make sure that the loops are not loose or the knot itself will not work. When tied correctly it can be very safe and useful knot and it is very easy to undo.

To make an Egg Loop knot:

1. Take the leader through a hook eye to bend it into a hook.
2. Make 20 wraps back toward bend in hook
3. Pull the end of the leader back through hook eye but in opposite direction and it needs to be tight. Make 5 wraps
4. Take the leader and pull it on to make sure that knot is tightened
5. Make a loop on top of the hook that can hold roe sack or eggs.

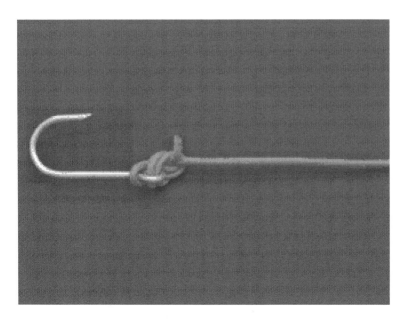

Palomar knot

Palomar knot is one of the strongest fishermen knots. It is used to ensure that the fishing line is attached to a hook or fly to a leader. With just a little practice, the Palomar knot can be tied in the dark. If tied properly, it is a hundred percent knot and it is impossible to pull out.

To make a Palomar knot:

1. Take the end of the loop and pull it through the eye of the hook.
2. Make overhand knot – needs to be loose – with the hook hanging from the bottom
3. While holding an overhand knot, pass that loop over the hook and slide it above the eye of the hook.

Tighten the knot down on the eye of the hook by pulling evenly the standing line and tag end.

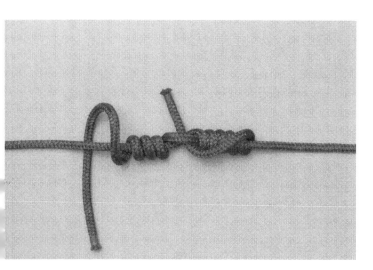

Blood Knot

The Blood Knot is a fishing knot and one of the favourite knots among fly fishermen. It is used for tying two lines together of the same or similar size. It is very easy to tie and to make sure to achieve better strength of the Blood knot it needs to have at least five and no more then seven wraps on each side of the center.

This knot also has great use in fly fishing, used to build a leader with the castable fly line on the bigger diameter end and the hook on the smaller one. The advantage of the Blood knot is that whichever way it is tightened, it makes symmetrical balance in the middle.

To make a Blood knot:

1. Band the ends of the line so that they are attached to each other.
2. Turn one end making five to seven wraps around the other end.
3. Take the teg end back through the lines.
4. Do the same action with the other end, making also between five and seven wraps in opposite direction.
5. Tighten the lines by pulling them away from each other.
6. Trim the ends.

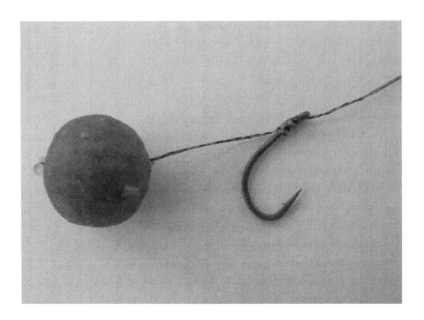

Hair rig

The hair rig will allow you to show but not actually put bait on the hook, allowing you to re-use it multiple times. It became immensely popular back in the 70s, and it got its name as fishermen used ponytail hair to make it. However, the material was later replaced by a braided thread as it wasn't as inconspicuous as needed, whereas the alternative was also more resistant and seldom lost.

To make a Hair rig:

1. Make a small overhand loop.
2. Slide the bait on the material of your choosing, followed by a bait stop through the loop so it doesn't fall off.
3. Take the hook link through the eye on the back (make sure to use enough hair material – it should never be shorter than the hook length).
4. Use the tag end to wrap the shank five times while holding the desired length of hair.
5. Pull the end through the hook eye on the back and tighten it.

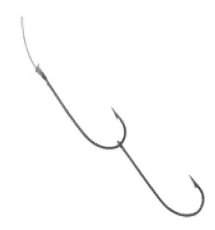

Stinger Hook

Stinger hook is an extra hook added to the current rig to prevent the less aggressive fish to bite short and snatch the bait. The short strikes will surely occur but with a stinger hook (which can be added to almost all hooks) set to trail the bait rig, creating a luring loop, you'll eliminate missing the short strikes.

To make a Stinger hook:

1. You'll need approximately a foot of monofilament line. Start by attaching the hook to the line – you can use Palomar knot here, as explained above, or any knot your prefer for that matter.
2. Make an overhand knot where you want your stinger hook to be, which should depend on the size of bait you use, and trim the line about half an inch above it (you can later use that end to tighten the hook).
3. Make a loop with the hook around the knot you've made, with the hook ending just under the loop when finished.
4. Take the set (stinger hook) in one hand and attach it to the jig – you can use the hook to pull the line behind through the look and it will slowly tighten while holding the tag end still outside the loop when it starts closing.
5. To remove the stinger, you should be able to simply pull the tag end to release it.

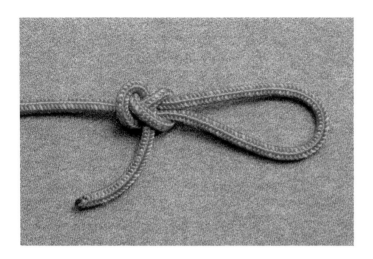

Angler's bend knot

An Angler's bend knot makes a locked loop. It is often used and holds quite well in bungy cord but his primary use was in creating an eye in fishing line. It won't slide under bungy cord if it is loaded and it will not untie once the load is off. It is a safe knot, but its disadvantage is that it does not bind very well, which can be a problem if the knot needs to be undone. Angler's bend knot can be tied either alone and the used or in combination with other knots and also can be tied to an object.

To make Angler's bend knot:

1. Create a loop at the end of the working line.
2. Create another loop at the top point of the first one but with the end going under the standing line.
3. Slide the tag end in between the loops.
4. Go with the top loop through the bottom loop.
5. Tie strongly the standing end and the loop by pulling and cut the end.

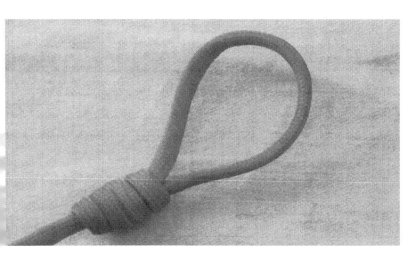

Surgeon's Loop Knot

The Surgeon's loop is another variation of the Double Overhand Knot which can be used to form a loop to loop connection or even allow the bait to move more naturally. Its main advantage, besides being reliable, is it's effortlessly and quickly tied at the end of a line. The loop is tied the same way as the Surgeon's Knot, whereas it can be easily tripled by adding an extra turn, but it will make the knot larger and not bring any additional gain.

To make a Surgeon's Loop Knot:

1. Make a bight at the end and tie it with an overhand knot.

2. Pass it through once more.

3. The loop size is then easily modifiable by adjusting the bight.

4. Tighten then knot by pulling.

5. Cut the loose end.

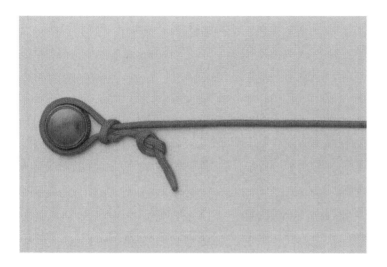

Arbor knot

The Arbor knot is used mostly by fishermen to join the fishing line to the fishing reel – spinning reel, bait casting reel or to the arbor. It is basically a noose knot. If the Arbor is available the easiest way to create the Arbor knot is my making the fixed noose knot and throwing on the Arbor and tying firmly. The point of creating this knot is to be safe that you have something strong enough that will hold in case you lose reel or rode and have to pull it by the line.

To make Arbor knot:

1. Take the end of the line and wrap it around the arbor of the spool.
2. With the same end create an Overhand knot around the standing part.
3. Continue with creating another Overhand knot in the tag end very close to the first Overhand knot.
4. Slip the overhand knot down by pulling the standing end, and then follow it with the second to jam together.
5. Cut the end.

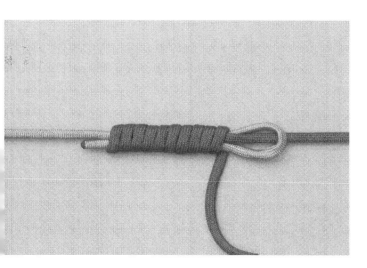

Albright knot

Albright knot or Albright special is used for attaching two lines of different width or material together, such as monofilament to braided line. It is famous knot among fishermen used for attaching two fishing lines together and it is also used for angling. It is a very secure knot, easily tied and it slides through guides when needed.

For Albright knot, it is very important to wrap the loops with precision around the initial loop of a larger line because it allows holding the loops under fingers while wrapping the line on.

To make Albright knot:

1. Create a loop in a heavier line.
2. Go with the end of a lighter line through that loop.
3. Continue by wrapping the end around itself and around that loop ten times.
4. Pull the end backward through the loop and against itself.
5. Tighten the knot firmly and cut the ends.

Chapter 6: Decorative Knots

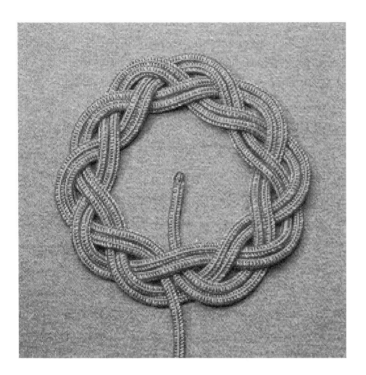

The Turk's Head

The Turk's Head is a decorative knot named after a turban for its likeness and used as an official part of scout uniform – usually as a woggle awarded for course completion. It's a closed loop made by interlocking rope strands, but usually not secured so the Turk's Head could actually be undone if needs be – used for starting a fire or similar tasks.

There are different variations to the knot, though, and it's generally regarded as a family of similar knots rather than a name for one, distinctive variation.

To make a simple Turk's Head:

1. Wrap a rope around your wrist.
2. Overlap and start interweaving.

3. Turn the rope as necessary for access.

4. Follow the process for all three turns.

5. Finish the knot by tucking or stitching the ends in.

It's important to note you can add variations on the simple knot to make it more distinctive and even unique.

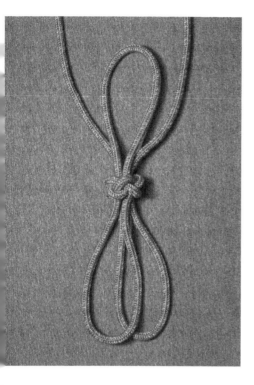

Fiador knot

The Fiador knot (also known as Theodore knot – a name supposedly corrupt after Theodore Roosevelt, just after the Spanish-American War) is a decorative knot used for different purposes such as halters, hops, and animal headgear. It's also known as Diamond knot, for obvious resemblance, and often referred to as a whole family of knots made with a single line and multiple loops into the knot. Considered very difficult to tie back in the day, it's said cowboys would take fees for making the Fiador knot.

To make the Fiador knot:

1. Make a loop on one end of the rope (so called L-shape).
2. Take the other end through it and then make another same, overlapping loop.
3. Take the loops (outer sides) and put them through the diamond in the middle.
4. Then pull the loops away toward ends.
5. Tighten slowly and carefully.

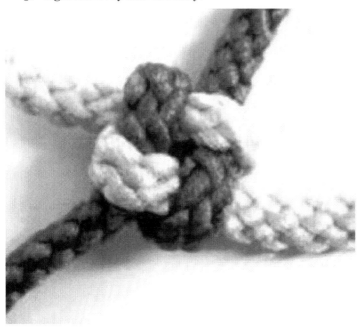

Lanyard knot

Lanyard knot (also known as the Knife Lanyard knot) forms a fixed decorative loop in the middle of a line, similar to the diamond knot in appearance and often used as a stopper on bracelets. While whether it's fashionable is questionable for some, it is very useful because of its size as one of the best such stoppers.

To make the Lanyard knot:

1. Make a bight.
2. Make a loop at one end of the rope.

3. Pull the other end of the rope under and around that loop (making a Carrick Bend).
4. Take this end on the outside the bight and through the centre of the Bend.
5. Repeat the same process with the other end.
6. Tighten the knot.

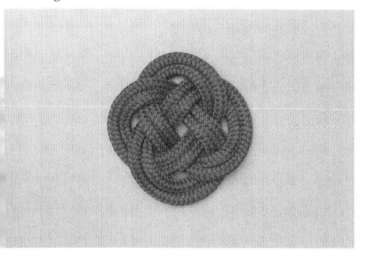

Celtic knot

Celtic knot is actually a family tree of decorative knots employing and representing Celtic and to a degree Christian style, often adapted and used in the ornamentation of monuments. There is a variation of patterns of different complexity, where experts can include squares, triangles, and even circles. The most common use for a Celtic knot nowadays are tablemats and hot pads, but we also find them in other decorative endeavors.

To make a simple Celtic knot:

1. Make an oval shaped loop.
2. Weave one end through the loop, first over the line then under.
3. Pass the line through the loop back to the start, using the same under and over sequence.
4. Follow the same path once more, using the same approach.

5. Tuck or stitch the ends in.

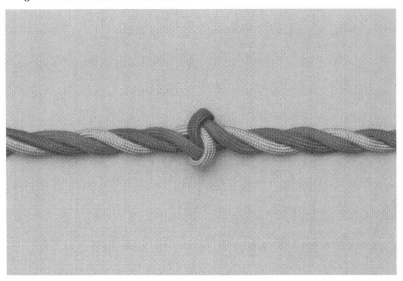

Wall knot

The Wall knot is a decorative knot made of strands, formerly used at the end of ropes fencing walkway leading on a ship, but now finds the best use in other combination knots. It's part of Wall and Crown knot, with great similarity to the Crown itself, differing only in the direction they're tied.

It is also often confused to the Turk's head, as it also employs a basket weave pattern. While it does look complicated, it's rather easy to make and it provides a small and, obviously, non-removable stopper knot as well as a beautiful decorative knot (part of Manrope Knot and the Matthew Walker knot).

To make a Wall knot:

1. You'll need to unwind the rope first (for decorative use best go halfway).
2. Take one strand around in the direction rope is laid and under the next.
3. Do the same with the second and the third strand.
4. The last strand should exit through the first one.
5. Tighten the knot.

6. Continue re-laying rope as it was.

Chapter 7: Other Knots

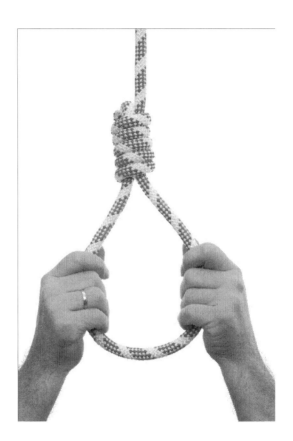

The Hangman's Noose

The hangman's noose is that knot that has been used for years by fishermen and boaters. It has also been used in hangings and lynchings (hence the term, hangman's noose). In many places it is considered a threatening gesture to have one displayed and is often illegal, but its not a difficult knot to make.

To make the Knot

1. Use a piece of cord or rope that is at least 3 ft long

2. Place the cord on a flat surface and form an "S" shape with the bottom or lead part of the cord left long, this is so you have something to tie it to when it's finished.

3. Compress the "S" shape of the cord until all three rows of it are nearly on top of each other, with only a few inches in between them.

4. Bunch the three lines of the cord tightly together in the middle until the ends look like a bow-tie.

5. Using the cord that made up the top, wrap it around, from the right side to the left, leaving about three to four inches of the cord unwrapped.

6. You should be left with a loop and a string on the left end, and just a loop on the right end of the "bow tie."

7. Poke the end of the cord through the top of the loop.

8. With your thumb to hold down the short piece of cord that you worked through the loop on the left-hand side so it bends over the loop.

9. Pull the right-hand side loop of the bow until it closes the loop on the left.

Adjust the noose until it's the size you want and the coils look nice and tight.

To make a Single Rope Knot Ladder

This simple knot ladder can be used as an emergency fire escape or as an aid for use in a child's tree house.

To make the Ladder

1. Place a single length of cord on a flat surface and form it into a "U" shape.

2. Take hold of the cord on the end of the right side of the "U" and slide your hand down the rope to measure out 1 foot (30 cm) of rope

3. Place the cord between your two hands and form it into an "S" shape. Then push the "S" down by bringing your hands together

4. To make the first row of your ladder, take the left end of the cord and thread it through the first, left bend of the "S." Bring the end of the cord under the bottom curve and wrap it around the whole "S" four times. Then feed the end of the cord

through the second, right bend of the "S" to secure the tie and complete the first rung.

5. Repeat this as many times as you need to create the ladder to your desired length

To Make a Rope Ladder With Wooden Rungs

1. First lay the cord flat on the ground, and make an overhand loop around 15 inches (38 cm) from the top-end.
2. Pull the standing part of the cord through the overhead loop, by putting your fingers through the underside of the loop, and grasping the standing part of the cord. Now, pull the standing part through the overhead loop. This should form a new loop.
3. Insert your wooden rung into the new loop and set it at the desired position, and tighten the rope. The knot should be visible above and below the rung
4. Tie an overhand knot by making an overhand loop, then passing the working end over, then through the loop. Ensure that the overhand knot is directly underneath the knot that is supporting the rung.
5. Repeat steps for the other piece of rope that will be used as the other side of the ladder. Taking care to make sure that your rungs are level and even.
6. The next rung should be started by placing the next overhand loop anywhere from 9 to 15 inches (23 to 38cm) from the previous wooden rung, it depends on the height of the people who may use the ladder, shorter distance for children and longer for adults The rungs should all be spaced uniformly, and distanced to suit those using it comfortably.
7. Keep going until you reach your desired length.
8. The ladder should be secured at the top using one of the knots described in the previous chapters such a timber hitch.
9. Securing the ladder at the bottom is optional, but securing it will greatly increase its stability and make it easier to climb.

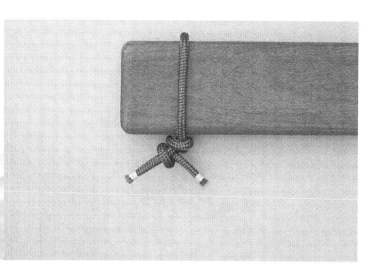

Butcher's knot

Butcher's knot is used in numerous situations. When tied it creates the first loop around the sack or pack. It is also used in preparing roasts or meat. When you make the first loop it shouldn't go down around the object. Its advantage is, when tightened correctly, its working end looks like a ring which makes it not so easy to untie.

Butcher's knot is so easy to tie and it can be done so fast that, observing professional butchers it is almost impossible to catching all the steps of it. It requires using very little string because knot can be created while its end is still attached to the coil. Butcher's knot is a knot when used for its purposes.

To make Butcher's knot:

1. Take the string and wrap it around the object.
2. At its standing end make an Overhand knot and pull firmly.
3. When you create the loop around your fingers, put the loop against the short end.
4. Take both ends and tie them strongly to create the knot.
5. Once done, cut the long end.

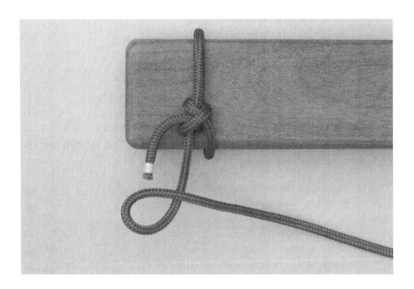

Corned beef knot

Corned beef knot – as its name says – is usually used as a binding knot for beef meat while it is prepared. It is often made in a smaller string or line. Due to the fact that beef meat often shrinks during preparation, the Corned beef knot needs to be tied at intervals and it will still hold in between while the meat is cooking.

To make Corned beef knot:

1. First, create the Buntline hitch and tie it firmly to the standing part.
2. Buntline needs to slide along the standing part so it will be tied in the process of preparation of meat.
3. After making sure that the beef is full shrunk go with the half hitch around the working end.

How to hogtie someone

To Hogtie someone correctly is not something anyone would normally do for fun as being tied in that position is usually very uncomfortable and not a pleasant experience to have, unless of course you are into kinky stuff and using soft restraints, but that's another story.

The most practical rope or cord to use to tie someone up is solid-braid nylon rope in 7/16″ or 3/8″ in diameter, these types of cord are available from most hardware or building supply stores. They, unlike many other types of cord or ropes have minimal stretch and the knots will stay easy to untie even after you pull them around.

Being hogtied, a person is totally incapacitated, with almost no chance of escape or even putting up any real resistance. When hogtied, a person's hands and feet are tied behind their back as well as being tied together, often with additional ties around the chest and thighs, most often the person is also gagged and blindfolded. It can be very dangerous to leave anyone unattended when hogtied, especially people who are elderly, overweight or unfit.

To make the hogtie

- The first step when you hogtie someone is to tie their hands behind their back, this can be done in several ways:
1. Tie the hands with the palms together this is the most comfortable for the victim.
2. Tie the hands with the wrists crossed and with the palms out, this is often uncomfortable for the victim.
3. Tie the arms together at the elbows behind the back and also secure the wrists. Often this is the most uncomfortable position, especially if the victim is large and overweight.
4. Wrap the cord around the wrists several times, then wrap it several times between the fingers and wrist, pull it tight and make a hitch knot.
5. If you want to secure the arms first (this is advisable if the victim is struggling) Tie the elbows by wrapping the cord several times around the arms just above the elbows and then several times between the lower arms and through the gape above the elbows, pull it tight and make a hitch knot. (Often, especially with large, overweight people it is not possible to bring their elbows together, behind

their backs because of physical limitations. In this event tie the elbows in the manner described for tying a rope handcuff as is explained in following knot description) Then tie the wrists either palm together or facing outwards.

6. In case you want to make the hogtie a little more secure when you tie the wrists pass the rope several times around the torso as well, and holding the arms in place, so the victim is unable to lift them up or down, secure the ropes with an overhand knot.

- Tie the feet by first removing the shoes and socks, then wrap the cord around the ankles several times, then through the gap above the ankles, between the legs and between the feet.

1. If the person is struggling, a good option is to first tie their legs together just under the knee, by wrapping the cord around their legs several times, then passing it between their lower legs and around and through the gap between their upper legs. If you apply pressure to the toes and fingers, especially against the normal movement of the joints, you can very quickly bring any captive to submission and control. The degree of pressure is determined by their amount of refusal to cooperate.

- The final step of applying the hogtie is to tie the wrists and ankles together behind the back. This is best done with a separate cord. First pass the cord through the ankle ties and then the wrist ties, pulling them together and bringing the ankles up by bending the person's knees. The ideal way to leave a person tied using this method is to have the soles of their feet facing you if you stand in front of them looking down their body. They can be left in this position or moved onto their side. In order to prevent the hogtie causing damage to the person and restricting the blood flow they should be constantly monitored.

To make a rope Handcuff

Rope handcuffs are quick and easy to make, there are several differences between handcuffing a willing partner for games and securing an unwilling person to restrict their movements. This description is for a willing partner, but the same principle applies to an un-willing or struggling person. If the handcuffs are for fun using soft linen or silk type rope or wrap is ideal, otherwise use solid-braid nylon rope of 7/16″ or 3/8″ in diameter

To make the Handcuff

About 25tf (8.5M) of cord is needed to make these handcuffs

- First have the person hold their hands about about 2 fist spaces apart
- Drape the cord over their wrists so there is an even overhang on each side
- Take the right side and wrap it around both the wrist 3 to 5 times and then take the left side and wrap it around the other way 3 to 5 times Warp both directions the same number of times). This will result in the victim's wrists being loosely wrapped.
- Bring the right and left cords under the wrists into the middle and cross them over each other in the center
- Then, starting with the right cord, wrap it tightly around the center between the wrists and continue winding or wrapping, moving the coils from the center to the outside or towards the wrists.
- Repeat with the left thread, winding or wrapping in the opposite direction from the center to the wrists.
- You should make an even number of coils or wraps on each side and finish when there is a small gap between the cord and the skin. Check to see if the knot is too tight or maybe too loose; adjust it by twisting each side in the direction you wound it to tighten or the other way to loosen.
- If you desire you can make several more turns or tie it off there.
- Lift the last loop on the right side and tuck the end of the cord through the resulting circle from inside to out. Repeat on the other side to finish tying it off, then pull on both ends of rope to make it secure.
- Any remaining cord can be cut off tucked in or used to tie the victim up to an activity area.

Conclusion

Thank you for reading my book Knot, Knots and More Knots, I hope you gained an insight on how to tie some of the more basic knots that are used in everyday life, tying your own knots is not as difficult as it at first seems. These knots were assembled because they have a proven track record of being safe, efficient and effective as well as being easy to tie. A small amount of practice and you will be able to tie a variety of knots for any situation you may encounter with the ease of a seasoned outdoors man.

Made in the USA
Middletown, DE
04 January 2019